BOOSTING YOUR MENTAL WELLBEING

BOOSTING YOUR MENTAL WELLBEING

10 minute steps for stressed healthcare professionals using CBT and mindfulness

LEE DAVID

MBBS, BSc, MRCGP, MA in cognitive behavioural therapy
GP and Cognitive Behavioural Therapist

DEBBIE BREWIN

OT, MSc CBT
Cognitive Behavioural Therapist, Supervisor and Trainer

Scion

© **Scion Publishing Ltd, 2023**

First published 2023

A CIP catalogue record for this book is available from the British Library.

ISBN 9781914961243

Scion Publishing Limited

The Old Hayloft, Vantage Business Park, Bloxham Road, Banbury OX16 9UX, UK

www.scionpublishing.com

Important Note from the Publisher

The information contained within this book was obtained by Scion Publishing Ltd from sources believed by us to be reliable. However, while every effort has been made to ensure its accuracy, no responsibility for loss or injury whatsoever occasioned to any person acting or refraining from action as a result of information contained herein can be accepted by the authors or publishers.

Readers are reminded that medicine is a constantly evolving science and while the authors and publishers have ensured that all dosages, applications and practices are based on current indications, there may be specific practices which differ between communities. You should always follow the guidelines laid down by the manufacturers of specific products and the relevant authorities in the country in which you are practising.

Although every effort has been made to ensure that all owners of copyright material have been acknowledged in this publication, we would be pleased to acknowledge in subsequent reprints or editions any omissions brought to our attention.

Registered names, trademarks, etc. used in this book, even when not marked as such, are not to be considered unprotected by law.

Cover design by Andrew Magee Design
Typeset by Evolution Design & Digital Ltd (Kent)
Printed in the UK

Last digit is the print number: 10 9 8 7 6 5 4 3

Contents

PART II Applying the GROWTH steps to common problems

Forewords

Not many healthcare professionals will go into healthcare believing that it is going to be an easy ride or a low stress career. Although we are taught how to treat and care for patients and need to pass multiple assessments and exams in the process, what we are not taught is how to look after our own health and wellbeing in the course of providing care to others.

The publication of this book is timely because currently it is difficult for those working in healthcare not to feel despondent about the future, when phrases such as "the NHS is in crisis", "record numbers of doctors retiring early", "NHS staff on strike again", and "I can't see my GP" are being bandied about in the news and on social media.

At NHS Practitioner Health, we look after many healthcare professionals who suffer with mental health and addiction problems. We do not just want our colleagues to survive their careers in healthcare but to thrive, and where better to start than ensuring we learn how to safeguard our own mental health. Healthcare professionals are notorious for putting the needs of others before their own, and we know from our work with the profession how this can so often lead to tragedy when our own basic needs are continually left unmet.

We are delighted that Lee David and Debbie Brewin have brought together their knowledge and experience in this book, to provide healthcare professionals with tools to facilitate better mental wellbeing and self-care. We would urge readers to put these tools into practice because good self-care takes work. With repetition such self-care will eventually become part of your day-to-day life and will ultimately lead to a healthier, happier you and therefore healthier, happier patients.

Dr Zaid Al-Najjar and Dr Helen Garr
Medical Directors, NHS Practitioner Health

This book could hardly have come at a better time. UK healthcare professionals across the spectrum are suffering. Suffering in so many different ways. Few thought that things could get worse as the Covid-19 pandemic receded, at least to an extent. But here we are in 2023 with a profession that many commentators have described as being 'on its knees'. Demand seems limitless, expectations unrealistic, and the workforce just doesn't have the capacity to offer satisfying consultations or healthcare experiences to all the patients seeking help for their health issues.

Debbie Brewin and Lee David bring a wealth of experience to this seemingly intractable problem – how do GPs look after themselves? GPs are unique in many ways. Their support is patchy at best. True, there are MDT meetings which play a role in providing patient care but also serve to support the healthcare professionals involved. Then there is the practice team, but with many of them direct employees of the GP partners, seeking help can involve challenging power structures within a practice. Unique among medical professionals, GPs spend long stretches of the day alone with their patients. This 'unsupervised practice' is not a feature of most secondary care provision. And it's a time when GPs can become isolated and lonely, carrying the seemingly impossible burdens of their patients with little direct help. Unlike therapists who can unburden during 'supervision sessions', this is rarely available to GPs and not funded as a structured support.

What this book does is to share a process which the authors call 'GROWTH' (read on). This goes much further than the unsatisfactory 'resilience training' and is underpinned by a strong background in CBT and ACT therapies. There is a clear message here about GPs needing to spend more time looking after themselves. Uniquely, this book provides a structure steeped in the theory of CBT and ACT on how overwhelmed GPs can regain control. And with this, can boost their mental wellbeing.

Professor Mark Ashworth
Professor of Primary Care, King's College London

About the authors

Lee David is a GP who works as a clinician and CBT therapist for NHS Practitioner Health, supporting health professionals coping with mental health difficulties. She has an interest in ACT, compassion and trauma therapy, and in working with people with neurodiversity. She also has a role in primary care education and is the director of 10 Minute CBT, which provides training for primary care health professionals to use realistic and effective brief CBT skills within routine consultations.

Debbie Brewin is a CBT, trauma and occupational therapist. She has worked in the NHS, social care and voluntary sector as a therapist, supervisor, trainer and clinical manager. Her special interests include work rehabilitation, wellbeing and personal growth. Alongside training, she has written manuals for clinical trials and presented at healthcare conferences in the UK and Europe.

Dedication

Lee and Debbie would like to dedicate this book to our NHS and to all the hard-working staff within it. We wish to thank them for their commitment and acknowledge the incredible care provided to patients throughout the service. We hope that this book provides a way to offer some care back to those professionals who may be in need of support in challenging times.

Introduction

- Do you feel motivated, enthusiastic and fulfilled at work, or are you feeling flat and aimless, counting down every second until it's time to go home?

- Can you remain calm and focused on the task at hand, or are you anxious, irritable or struggling to prioritise and maintain your energy?

- Do you stay resilient and reflective when things don't go to plan, or can you get overwhelmed or react defensively when facing challenges or feeling criticised?

- Would you benefit from finding ways to maximise your wellbeing and energy and promote personal **GROWTH**? Keep reading…

Why read this book?

Primary care is one of the most challenging fields of healthcare. With 90% of patient consultations taking place in general practice, the pressure is intense. High levels of demand and complexity, a dense workload, long hours, and the emotional toll of the job leave clinicians vulnerable to distress and mental health challenges. These difficulties have been compounded by Covid as we cope with practical and political pressures through and beyond the pandemic.

As a health professional you have high levels of knowledge and skills in supporting wellbeing in your patients, but how often do you apply this to your own physical and emotional needs?

This book contains a practical toolkit for all clinicians, particularly those working in primary care. It includes a series of bite-sized skills to help you:

- Improve the balance between different parts of your life.

- Learn to make yourself a priority, take better care of yourself, and refuel before hitting 'empty'.

- Find ways to thrive and regain your enjoyment and enthusiasm for work and life.

- Make positive or helpful choices when struggling with difficult thoughts and feelings.

- Discover new strategies for dealing with stress, low mood and anxiety, and for coping with challenging situations such as complaints, change and unrealistic workload demands.

Some case stories

Kabir, Salaried GP: *"I used to love the job, but now I just can't stand the thought of going into work. I dread it and I wake up on Monday mornings feeling sick at the thought of going into the surgery…"*

Kabir had always wanted to be a GP and previously found work enjoyable and satisfying. However, more recently he has found it increasingly difficult to motivate himself to get into work each day. He struggles with concentration and his energy levels are low. He feels exhausted and cannot find pleasure in things he used to enjoy. He has given up most of his usual leisure activities such as regular visits to the gym.

Janet, Nurse Practitioner: *"I have always been thorough and conscientious at work. Recently, I've been getting preoccupied and worried that I might miss something or make a terrible mistake at work. It's hard to think about anything else. Even when I'm with my family, I find myself thinking about work and whether I've done everything correctly…"*

Janet is having difficulty recovering after a recent complaint. No major harm came to the patient, and she was well supported by colleagues, but she found it extremely distressing, and has lost confidence in her abilities. Janet has recurrent intrusive worries that she might miss something or that another patient might complain about her, and how terrible this would be. She's also highly self-critical and feels inner shame and embarrassment about the mistake that occurred.

Janet used to enjoy working with her colleagues but has recently started to wonder if she really has what it takes to do the job. She takes great pains to hide all her possible shortcomings for fear she might be 'found out' and then rejected. This means she is working longer hours and is finding it increasingly difficult to keep the balance with her family life.

All the examples in this book are fictional but are based on our own experiences of the reality of working in primary care. We will come back to meet Kabir, Janet and many others, throughout the book, to find out how each individual coped with their difficulties.

Stress and pressure in primary care

Many factors contribute to stress, burnout and mental health difficulties in primary care health professionals (Walker *et al.*, 2019). These include:

- Long hours and an intense workload, balancing time pressures with effective decision-making, patient safety, and maintaining relationships with patients and colleagues amidst the increasing complexity of patient care.

- Growing demands for access including telephone, email and face-to-face contact, alongside unrealistic patient expectations or hostile comments from politicians and the press.

- Adapting systems and practices to cope with frequent change and moving goalposts.

- The emotional toll of general practice which involves caring for people with psychosocial problems and emotional distress, and managing anxious, abusive and confrontational patients or colleagues.

- Fear of mistakes, complaints or litigation. Coping with a complaint places clinicians at a higher risk of burnout and mental health problems, with the level of distress increasing in relation to complaint severity (Bourne *et al.*, 2016).

- Experiencing professional isolation, fragmentation of practice teams or a lack of support.

- Difficulties with recruitment and understaffing.

- Dealing with regulatory demands and keeping up to date, including practice inspections, appraisals and revalidation.

- Moral distress and conflict with health professionals' personal values if we are unable to meet patient needs due to limitations in practice systems or the wider health service.

Reluctance to seek help

Mental health problems are common in health professionals, yet there are often delays in seeking help and appropriate treatment. Continuing to work whilst suffering from a mental health difficulty is high among doctors, who tend to under-report illness and take one-third fewer sick days than other healthcare workers (Murphy, 2014).

There are many reasons why a clinician may be unwilling to seek help for mental health problems. We may fear that having a mental health problem will be perceived as a sign of incompetence or weakness, have concerns about lack of confidentiality, or have a strong sense of duty to our patients. Understaffing and a lack of cover can also make it harder to take time off when needed.

Effective care for mental health is essential for health professionals. If unrecognised, these may affect our concentration, productivity and decision-making. Clinicians who work whilst experiencing mental health difficulties are more likely to develop long-term problems, and it can also affect patient care, with an increased risk of medical errors and adverse patient outcomes (Kinman and Teoh, 2018).

Warning signs

We will talk in more detail throughout the book about how to recognise stress, burnout and mental health difficulties, but here are some pointers for possible problems in you or your colleagues:

Are you experiencing any of the following?	Have you noticed this?
Working more slowly or finding it harder to get through tasks than previously or compared to colleagues	
Finding it harder to make decisions or prioritise tasks	
Irritability with colleagues or patients	
Emotional outbursts or over-sensitivity to possible criticism or negativity from others	
Becoming rigid and inflexible, defensive, and finding it difficult to compromise or see the perspective of others	
Arriving early and leaving late, yet still struggling with workload, particularly if compared with colleagues	
Frequent lateness or unexplained absences during the working day	
Taking frequent sick leave	
Avoiding asking for help or support when it is needed, particularly in juniors or trainees	
Problems with exams, appraisal or revalidation procedures	
Feelings of uncertainty and disillusionment with medicine or primary care	

Responding to the challenges

Working in primary care can be stressful, yet can also be incredibly meaningful, rewarding and enjoyable. Health professionals are often busy and juggling multiple priorities, but if we take a little time to reflect, it may be possible to reconnect with some of the positive aspects of our role.

How we respond to all the challenges is likely to affect our mood and mental health. Exhausted clinicians may slip into negative spirals of unhelpful coping strategies such as over-working, having difficulty switching off, and not making time for rest, recuperation or other wellbeing activities.

In this book we will highlight some key skills that support individuals to thrive in their work and personal lives. Making time to prioritise choices that promote wellbeing is realistic and achievable, and making small changes in multiple life areas can have a surprisingly significant cumulative impact on mood. Alongside personal self-care strategies, it may also be important to work towards organisational and political changes that optimise working conditions and support clinician mental health.

10 minute steps to GROWTH

In the book, we will introduce you to six 10 minute steps leading to positive mental health, wellbeing and personal **GROWTH**. These are derived from theoretical backgrounds including cognitive behavioural therapy, behavioural activation, compassion-focused therapy, acceptance and commitment therapy, and mindfulness.

Here is a quick overview of the steps that we'll be looking at throughout this book:

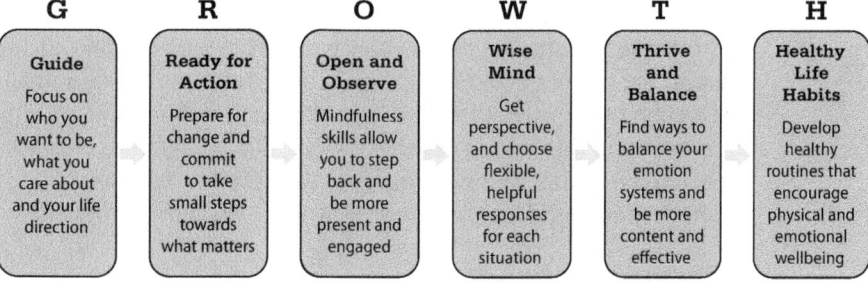

G	**R**	**O**	**W**	**T**	**H**
Guide Focus on who you want to be, what you care about and your life direction	**Ready for Action** Prepare for change and commit to take small steps towards what matters	**Open and Observe** Mindfulness skills allow you to step back and be more present and engaged	**Wise Mind** Get perspective, and choose flexible, helpful responses for each situation	**Thrive and Balance** Find ways to balance your emotion systems and be more content and effective	**Healthy Life Habits** Develop healthy routines that encourage physical and emotional wellbeing

These steps don't have to be followed in order – and some might be more relevant to you than others. You might also need to go back and forth between steps several times, especially with complex or stressful situations.

Throughout the book we will invite you to:

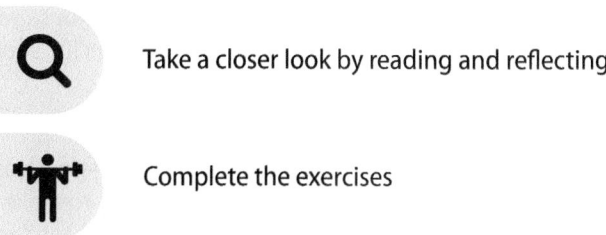

Take a closer look by reading and reflecting

Complete the exercises

Write down your thoughts

 Set a realistic goal or a target

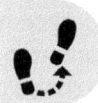 Take an action step

Follow your inner guide

 This involves making decisions and choosing actions that have personal meaning, a wider purpose, and are important to you. Your **Guide** acts as an inner compass, which points in the direction of your most important values and helps you see the big picture and choose which direction to take. You might ask yourself questions like: Who and what do I care about most? What kind of person do I want to be? What do I want to stand for – in my professional and my personal life?

Ready for action

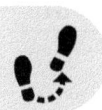 Being **Ready for Action** is a behavioural skill which involves making active choices about what we do and how we react to the changing circumstances and situations of our lives. It's often helpful to focus on taking small steps in the direction of our values, or important life goals. At times, these decisions may be clear, and the choices may be obvious, but when facing uncertainty, we may need to be flexible and experiment with different strategies, taking notice of what happens and learning from experience to guide us forwards.

Open and observe

 We will introduce some brief mindfulness skills that we can bring into our busy lives, helping to improve our awareness and self-understanding, manage challenging emotions, and find ways to appreciate the moment. Learning to **Open and Observe** might involve taking a moment to check in with yourself, notice your thoughts, feelings and urges. You can then step back to make room for uncomfortable thoughts and feelings without getting caught up or dominated by them. This creates a space in which we can choose which actions are likely to be helpful in the context of our life and the specific situation.

Engage your wise mind

 Our mind is our inner voice and includes our thoughts, beliefs, ideas, expectations, memories and personal stories. It enables us to make complex decisions and plans and can be an incredibly powerful and useful tool. But at

other times, our mind can be critical and unhelpful, producing thoughts which are self-limiting, and which affect our feelings and actions in negative ways.

Using **Wise Mind** may involve taking a short pause to expand your perspective and reflect on how to approach challenging circumstances. You may need to step back and 'unhook' from unhelpful, critical or negative thinking patterns that may be keeping you stuck, draining your confidence, and making it harder to perform effectively. Instead, you can learn to recognise helpful thoughts that direct you towards your values and allow these to guide your actions and choices.

Thrive and balance

In this chapter we will explore some of the triggers for stress, and how the 'three circles model' provides a simple way to understand how our brain, nervous system and emotions interact and influence how we function as a whole. In **Thrive and Balance** we will explore ways to thrive emotionally and achieve optimal performance and wellbeing, by finding a balance between the systems:

- **Threat** emotions alert us to potential danger and urge us to take action to stay safe. Overuse of the threat system can lead to anxiety, stress and irritability, as we live with an exaggerated sense of danger and risk.

- **Drive** emotions act to energise and excite us, helping us pay attention to opportunities and achieve goals. Overuse of the drive system can lead to excessive striving, exhaustion and addiction. If the drive system becomes linked with the threat system, it can also lead to self-criticism and fear of failure.

- **Calm and connect system** helps us experience feelings of contentment, safety and self-compassion. This system is sensitive to closeness and bonding with others and helps us recover when facing problems or when things go wrong.

Healthy life habits

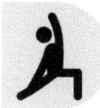

Building **Healthy Life Habits** involves finding ways to maximise our physical and emotional wellbeing. This involves making choices about our daily routines and patterns of living that support this, including being physically active, eating well, maintaining a healthy body weight, getting enough sleep, cutting back on unhealthy choices such as limiting alcohol or technology habits, and taking care of long-term conditions and physical illness.

How to use this book

Part I of this book includes exercises and activities to help you practise and learn more about each of the 10 minute **GROWTH** steps. It is helpful to read through these chapters in order before moving onto the second part of the book.

Part II focuses on applying the steps to some of the common difficulties that we may experience in primary care. These can be read in any order – start with the chapters that seem most relevant to you! Some of the important topics we will cover in this section include:

- Personality traits and traps such as perfectionism, imposter syndrome and being a 'chronic hero' that can make us more prone to mental health challenges

- Overcoming low mood, low motivation and burnout, if you are trying to 'drink from an empty cup'

- Coping with anxiety, uncertainty and worry, perhaps if you are training, taking exams or feeling overwhelmed with constant change

- Managing change and loss, developing flexibility in relation to life's inevitable changes and supporting the process of grief and acceptance

- Strengthening important relationships, setting boundaries and navigating tricky encounters with others

- Surviving significant life events: coping with loss, trauma and when things go wrong, such as complaints and errors at work.

Back to the case stories

Let's go back to the two individuals that we met at the beginning of this chapter and think how they might use the 10 minute **GROWTH** steps to work on their wellbeing.

Kabir, Salaried GP: *"I used to love the job, but I had got to the point where I just couldn't stand the thought of going into work. I would dread it and used to wake up on Monday mornings feeling sick at the thought of going into the surgery…"*

Applying the 10 minute GROWTH steps:

- **Guide** – Kabir might start by turning to his inner **Guide** to help him focus on his personal values and reconnect with his motivation for working.

- **Ready for Action** – he might then get **Ready for Action**, setting himself some small, realistic goals that move him towards valued life areas, which may help to lift his mood and sense of achievement. He might focus on getting back to the gym or something easier to achieve such as a regular walk with friends or family, so that he feels connected and supported and regains some motivation.

- **Open and Observe** – Kabir could also learn to use **Open and Observe** skills to step back from difficult emotions.

- **Wise Mind** – he could also engage his **Wise Mind** to seek a wider perspective.

- **Thrive and Balance** – his **Wise Mind** could help him to make choices that allow him to **Thrive** by creating more **Balance** between his emotion systems.

- **Healthy Life Habits** – Kabir might also reflect on whether any personality traits may be slipping into unhelpful traps, which prevent him from creating sustainable **Healthy Life Habits**. He may benefit from turning to *Chapter 8* to understand more about how to overcome negative cycles of behaviour and emotion in low mood and depression.

Janet, Nurse Practitioner: *"I've always been conscientious and thorough in my work but lately I've been getting overwhelmed by worries that I might miss something or make a terrible mistake. Even when I'm with my family, I find myself thinking about work and whether I've done everything correctly…"*

Applying the 10 minute GROWTH steps:

- **Guide** – Janet might need to remind herself about her personal values and connect with her inner **Guide** which may prioritise reconnecting with her family, and not allowing worry about work to get in the way of personal relationships.

- **Ready for Action** – she could choose to take small actions that are in line with her core values.

- **Open and Observe** – she could also use **Open and Observe** skills to help manage her worry and distress, and to ground her in the present moment, so she is able to pay more attention and focus on enjoying time with her family.

- **Wise Mind** – using this will help her step back and gain perspective on the mistake, and she may also benefit from developing her sense of self-compassion to counter the distress and shame that often arises when things have gone wrong.

- **Thrive and Balance** – Janet may find it helpful to think about ways to create balance in her life, and step out of cycles of rumination and worry, helping to reduce her sense of stress and overwhelm at work.

- **Healthy Life Habits** – reflecting on her individual personality traits may also help encourage sustainable **Healthy Life Habits** and minimise any personality traps that are keeping her stuck. She might also wish to look at *Chapter 11* which explores ways of coping after significant life events, setbacks and challenges.

Don't just read this book – try it out!

We learn new skills by actively testing out new ideas, then noticing what happened, adjusting and repeating. So, we would encourage you to try out these skills and experiment to find out how you might bring any new ideas into your life. Then repeat the steps until you have developed a new, healthy habit.

Little and often

It often helps to find a little bit of space on a regular basis to focus on yourself and what you need to live and work optimally. Spending a short time regularly reading and practising the techniques in this book is likely to have the greatest benefit. You will be surprised at what you can achieve in just 10 minutes!

Keep a record

It's easier to remember what you have learnt when you write it down. You can use this book, a journal, a computer or your phone to keep track of your thoughts and reflections, and any important insights or helpful tips. This will also help you to notice whether your feelings change as you progress through the book.

EXERCISE: What brings you here?

What made you pick up this book and start reading? What is your 'story'? Life often does not run smoothly, and many of us are facing multiple different challenges and difficulties. Getting it down on paper, or on the computer – anywhere but inside your head – can be a cathartic process that helps make sense of what you are dealing with.

Make a note of your thoughts

What problems are you coping with at the moment? What are your major challenges?

What would you most like to change or improve in your life? What would make you feel more enthusiastic, empowered, energetic or excited to go to work? Does this seem realistic or like an impossible dream?

How will you know if things are improving? What would you or other people notice? What might be the first thing to tackle?

What would you be doing differently if you felt better about your life or your work? What actions would you take?

Seek help if you need it

Do seek support if you are struggling. Help is available and can make a huge difference to enable you to overcome emotional challenges and difficulties with your mental health.

There are many different options. You might talk to a friend, a colleague, to a family member or your own GP. There are also a variety of support organisations that you can turn to, and we have included links to some key sources of help in the resources section of the book.

It's essential for us as clinicians and health professionals to be willing to stand up for ourselves and access the support and treatment that can enable us to thrive in our personal and working lives.

Summary

This introduction covered the concepts behind the **GROWTH** steps to wellbeing in primary care:

- **Guide** – know who you want to be, what you care about and your life direction

- **Ready for Action** – prepare for change and take small steps towards what matters

- **Open and Observe** – learn to be present, aware, and able to step back and make space for difficult thoughts and emotions without being overwhelmed

- **Wise Mind** – gain perspective, choose helpful responses and do what works best in the circumstances

- **Thrive and Balance** – use the three circles model to balance your emotion systems and be more content and effective

- **Healthy Life Habits –** develop healthy routines that encourage physical and emotional wellbeing.

Final thoughts

What did you find most helpful, interesting or surprising in this chapter?

Set a target

In the end it's not what you read or watch or listen to, it's what you put into action that counts. What would you most like to get out of this book?

Can you commit to reading this book and spending time on yourself for 10 minutes each day? Anything else?

Take an action step

What are your next steps? How can you bring this into your daily life in a small way?

Writing it down will help you remember. It will also help you to commit to doing something differently.

What I am going to do now:

01 Follow your inner Guide

- Do you have a clear sense of who you are, what you need, and the direction in which your life is headed?

- Do you take time to reflect on what's most important, or do you feel confused, uncertain or dissatisfied with your life?

- Are you able to keep a balance between competing priorities, or do you spend too long on activities that don't provide much sense of purpose or pleasure?

- Do you want to focus more on what really matters to you? Keep reading...

1.1 What do we mean by your inner Guide?

Your inner **Guide** acts like a beacon or a pathfinder, providing purpose and direction, and helping you to focus on what matters most. It can help you make decisions and choose actions that are more likely to help you manage your stress. It also helps you to feel fulfilled and contented.

Using your **Guide** involves:

- Thinking about your **values**, the 'bigger picture'

- Discovering what is important to you and what gives your life **meaning** and **purpose**

- Understanding what motivates you, and your unique, personal **needs** and **desires**

- Prioritising **actions** that take you in the direction you wish your life to go, even if this involves effort and overcoming challenges.

PAUSE AND REFLECT: What matters to you?

You have been granted a generous paid sabbatical from practice for six months… What would you choose to do?!

Imagine having a fully paid sabbatical from work. Your financial pressures are gone, and you have complete freedom to decide what to do during this period.

Spend 2–3 minutes thinking: What would you do with your time? Who would you do it with? Why would you choose to do these things? What types of activity are most important to you?

Make a note of your thoughts here:

Anthony, GP Partner: "Over the past year or so I feel like I've lost track of 'me' – it's as if I don't know who I am or what I want to do with my time. I feel like I'm just going through the motions, and I feel quite numb and empty."

Anthony has been a full-time GP Partner for over 10 years. He used to enjoy the job, and had an active life outside work, playing tennis and swimming regularly and spending time with his family. Over the past year, work has been increasingly busy, and it has been hard to recruit new staff. Anthony has found himself working longer hours and cutting back on many of the activities he used to enjoy. It's harder to motivate himself to go to work each day and when he gets home, it's usually late in the evening so his kids are already asleep, and he rarely gets to see his family before heading to bed himself.

Feeling numb and empty suggests that Anthony has become disconnected from what really matters to him. The starting point for improving his wellbeing is to reconnect with his inner Guide, which can remind him what he genuinely cares about and what is most important in his life. This can help Anthony to start to make active choices about how to prioritise his limited time each day. As he takes small, realistic steps towards his Guide and his core personal values, he may find that his mood starts to lift as he gets more meaning and enjoyment from his life.

1.2 Finding your values

Following your inner **Guide** involves recognising your personal values. Values are like an internal compass which help to give your life a meaningful direction, by pointing in the direction of the people and activities that you care about most deeply. The first step towards finding your values involves asking yourself some 'big' questions such as:

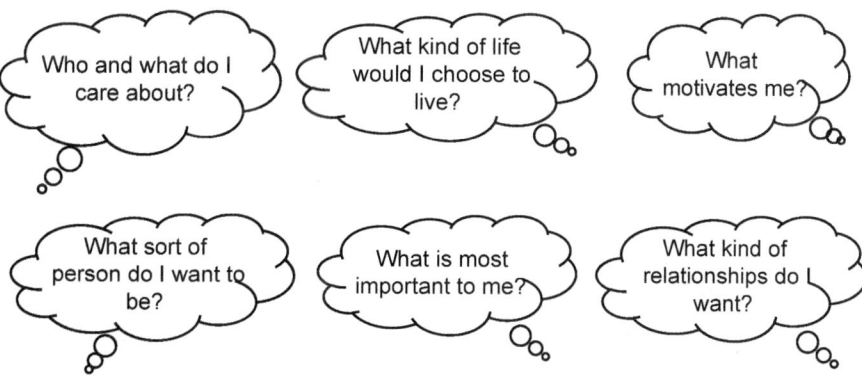

Who and what do I care about?

What kind of life would I choose to live?

What motivates me?

What sort of person do I want to be?

What is most important to me?

What kind of relationships do I want?

EXERCISE: Use the following table to help identify your values

What gives your life meaning and purpose – at home and at work?	
How do you feel when you are involved in an activity that is meaningful to you?	
Choose one or more activities that you do regularly, such as exercise, going to work, or a regular hobby, and ask yourself: What motivates you to do this? Why is it important to you?	

Why do values matter?

We know that many clinicians are feeling exhausted by the pressures and stresses of balancing a busy home life with demands at work and other responsibilities. Your values can help you choose how to live, even when life is tough, when things are going wrong, or when the challenges may seem insurmountable. In fact, this is exactly when it may be most important to engage and live most fully according to your values. When you are feeling stressed, anxious or stuck, you can turn to your inner **Guide** to help you to motivate and inspire yourself to make helpful choices and to keep going in the face of life's difficulties.

Knowing your values can help you to make purposeful decisions that are consistent with who you want to be as a person. If you value being a loving, caring parent, it's worth making the effort to take time to engage with your family after a busy day at work. If you value closeness and connection in your relationships at work, it's worth making the effort to have lunch or a coffee break with colleagues, rather than simply 'pushing through' and ignoring your need for interaction.

Values checklist

Let's remind ourselves about some of the key facts about values and our inner **Guide**:

Values are...	Values are not...
✔ Values are directions not destinations: values focus on the journey and the route that we travel, not the outcome	✖ Values are not goals or milestones to achieve, or actions to tick off our to-do list
✔ Values are flexible principles which evolve over time with changing circumstances and priorities	✖ Values are not fixed or rigid rules about what we 'should' or 'must' do, or what's 'wrong', 'right', 'good' or 'bad'
✔ Our values reflect the kind of person we want to be and the personal qualities we value in ourselves and others	✖ Following our values is not always easy and may involve making difficult choices or experiencing uncomfortable feelings
✔ Values involve looking at the big picture, with a perspective that extends beyond ourselves	✖ Recognising our values does not make us self-centred and does not involve focusing only on ourselves or on one specific goal
✔ Values represent our individual choices, and may be similar, overlapping or completely different from the people around us or in our culture	✖ It's not necessary to conform to other people's values or opinions, without acknowledging or taking into account our own beliefs and perspectives

EXERCISE: What are your values?

Take a few minutes to look at the following list of values. Some may apply to your professional life and others may be more relevant to your personal life.

Try to rate how important each value is to you on a scale of 1–5 (where 1 is not very important, and 5 is extremely important). Aim for around 4–6 values that are very important (scoring 4 or 5) to you at the moment.

It may be difficult to choose your values, or to be certain which are most important. Just pick the values which seem to be most relevant for now. You can evolve and amend your choices later if needed.

Values	How important? (1–5)		How important? (1–5)
ACHIEVEMENT: making progress towards important professional and personal goals		**FREEDOM:** finding space and reducing restrictions and demands in your life	
ACTIVE: participating in physical activities, exercise, movement or sports		**FUN:** humour, laughter and enjoyment	
ADVENTURE: having new and exciting experiences		**INDIVIDUALITY:** expressing yourself as a unique person, celebrating diversity and difference	
ASPIRE: thinking about the future and finding opportunities to grow and develop		**INTIMACY:** close personal and/or sexual relationships	
AUTONOMY: being independent and able to make decisions and choices		**LEADERSHIP:** taking responsibility for guiding others and making choices	
BELONGING: feeling accepted within a group, community, team, organisation, culture or a loving family		**NATURE:** the outdoors, animals and the natural world	

BODY and HEALTH: taking care of your body, health and appearance		**ORGANISATION:** being prepared, following, or developing patterns or routines	
CALM: finding a sense of peace and tranquillity in your life		**PROFESSIONALISM:** maintaining high standards of conduct, relationships and practice	
CARE: receiving and offering care and support to colleagues, patients, family and friends		**PROGRESS:** embracing change and personal or professional development	
COMPASSION: offering acceptance, kindness and empathy to ourselves and others		**RESPECT:** giving and receiving acknowledgement and respect	
CONNECTION: experiencing love, closeness and affection with important people in your life		**SPIRITUALITY and RELIGION:** upholding personal beliefs, traditions and practices	
CONTRIBUTION: offering time and expertise, professionally or personally, in a way that feels meaningful to you		**TEAMWORK:** working within a group, supporting each other with shared objectives	
CREATIVITY: expressing or appreciating creativity in diverse ways, including music, literature and art		**VARIETY:** seeking out new and varied experiences	
ETHICS: acting with a sense of integrity, honesty and fairness		**WORLD MATTERS:** politics, global or environmental issues	
FINANCE: having sufficient income, financial security and stability		**Other important values?** List these here:	

PAUSE AND REFLECT: Finding your values

Did you find it straightforward or challenging to prioritise your values?	
What was difficult? Was it hard to limit your choices, or did none of the values seem quite right?	
Are your values balanced? For example, do you have a balance of responsibility and relaxation? Or a balance between values at work and at home?	
Are there any values that are important, but that you have neglected recently?	
Are there any values that seem overwhelming, or are becoming a pressure or a demand? Can you find any ways to hold these more lightly or flexibly?	

Let's return to Anthony, who has been feeling disconnected from his values and has lost motivation at work…

Anthony completes the Values exercise. At first, he found it hard to connect with what motivated him at work, as he felt so fed up and low. After some thought, he answered:

*"I think what has always motivated me at work is a sense of **contribution**. I like being able to contribute to my patients and my colleagues. I also enjoy the **variety** that we have in primary care."*

We also asked Anthony to think about what activities he used to enjoy and how life might be different if he started to feel brighter:

"I used to love sport. I did all kinds of different sports at university, but I particularly enjoyed tennis and swimming. I haven't had time to do those for at least a year now."

To find Anthony's values, we asked him what he enjoys most about sport. Is it physical activity and fitness, connecting with friends through sport, caring for his body, or a sense of achievement when he wins a match?

Anthony recognised that he particularly valued the camaraderie and banter from playing tennis with friends, and he also enjoyed having a peaceful space away from work when he went swimming.

*"My values are **connection** with other people and a sense of **freedom** from all the jobs and demands. I also really value how it feels in my **body** to be more fit and active. Having some personal **space** and **autonomy** also seems important – some time alone. I can see how I have lost touch with some of my values almost completely in the past year."*

1.3 Living your values

A value is a general life direction that doesn't have a defined endpoint. You can't tick values such as 'respect', 'autonomy' or 'compassion' off your to-do list, but you can plan and carry out actions that relate to each of these values. If your value is education, then a goal may be to read a book, achieve a qualification or pass an exam. For a value such as security, your goal could be to buy your own home, find a new job or achieve a promotion at work.

So, now that you have met your inner **Guide**, the next step is to plan '**towards actions**' which move you in the direction of important values. For example, you might choose to go for a walk if your value is physical health or activity. This action might also take you towards other important values such outdoors, self-care or – if you walk with a friend – connection.

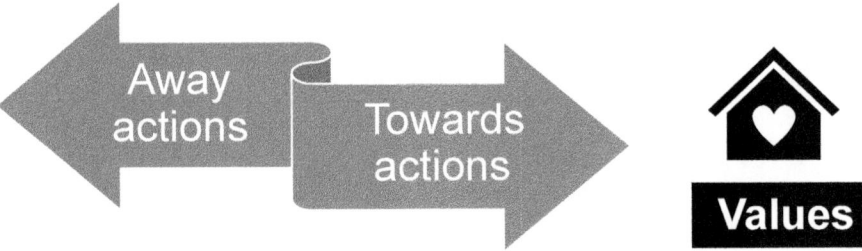

Taking a Towards action often involves overcoming some short-term emotional or physical discomfort, but it reaps the benefit of being fulfilled and true to yourself in the long term. Choosing to go out for a walk may involve overcoming a sense of apathy or fatigue, or you may have to pull yourself away from other activities such as zoning out in front of the TV.

In contrast, an Away action moves you away from the things you care about. Examples include not going out to meet a friend you care about because you feel too low or anxious, or not getting an important task done because you've been hooked into mindlessly surfing social media on your phone.

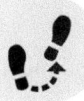

TAKE ACTION

In *Chapter 2* we look in more detail at setting goals and planning actions. For now, can you think of just one small action that would take you towards an important value? Write it here:

We asked Anthony whether he could think of a really small step in the direction of one of his values.

"Trying to plan a game of tennis seems overwhelming. But I could try to find my tennis shoes in the garage. Maybe I could have a look at the times that our local court is open, as I could take my daughter there to hit the ball with me for a short while at the weekend."

Anthony wasn't sure that this would be enough to make a difference in his life. And of course, this is just the first small step. What's important is that this is a step towards one of his personal and meaningful values.

1.4 Recognising your needs

Finding ways to recognise and meet your important needs is another way to help you follow your inner **Guide**. Values and needs are similar in many ways and may overlap, but there are also some important differences.

Values refer to long-term, core priorities about what we find meaningful and important in life. Needs represent the immediate urges or impulses that influence us in the context of one particular situation. Needs tend to be universal to most human beings. They range from basic needs such as food, shelter, rest and security, through to emotional needs such as the need for love and acceptance, or for space and autonomy.

Needs are dynamic, like a short-term pattern of changing weather. Thinking about your needs involves noticing what's going on for you right now, in the present moment, rather than reflecting on past patterns, your identity or long-term goals. Understanding your needs can help you decide on your priorities and can help to set realistic goals that move you towards long-term values.

Your needs matter

The bottom line is that your needs matter, and as a health professional, you must recognise and take care of your own needs before trying to care for others. This is a classic example of putting on your own oxygen mask first.

We live and work in busy, hectic environments, with multiple competing needs and priorities, which are dynamic and changing. It's impossible to meet every single one of our needs at all times. But starting to recognise and meet our essential needs, as best we can, in the circumstances we are in, is the key to wellbeing.

So, if your goal is to pass a professional exam, your long-term values may involve education and personal achievement. And as you make a decision each evening about how to use your precious time, you may need to weigh up your differing needs: Should you study? Spend time with your family? Cook a nutritious meal? Or take time to relax and sleep?

Weighing up decisions involving needs and values will depend on many factors including how soon the exam is, how hungry or tired you are, whether activity might help you to focus and concentrate, and whether your dog needs exercise… The balance of competing needs will vary over time, so you may need to take a flexible approach that takes personal wellbeing and the big picture into account to help you decide what's helpful on any particular occasion.

Understanding and noticing our different needs

The box below includes some of the common human needs. This is not an exhaustive list and may differ from person to person. You can add any of your own important needs below:

Important human needs

- **Acceptance:** empathy, love, respect, support, approval

- **Acknowledgement:** to matter, to be valued, appreciated, heard, seen, to have respect, recognition, mourning

- **Autonomy:** choice, independence, freedom, power, responsibility, space, being empowered, consent

- **Belonging:** communication, community, cooperation, inclusion, participation, sharing

- **Connection:** affection, appreciation, closeness, warmth, care, partnership

- **Enjoyment:** fun, play, laughter, excitement, celebration, humour

- **Essential physical care:** food, water, shelter, air, sleep, rest, health, movement

---

- **Inspiration:** beauty, faith, hope, peace, presence
- **Meaning and purpose:** contribution, effectiveness, fulfilment, achievement, using skills, creativity
- **Safety and security:** financial and physical safety, predictability, consistency and dependability
- **Sense of self:** authenticity, integrity, self-acceptance and self-compassion, dignity
- **Trust:** honesty, equality, fairness, certainty, loyalty
- **Understanding:** awareness, clarity, learning, discovery, growth, stimulation, exploration
- **Any other important needs:**

Yasmine, Practice Nurse: *"It was an incredibly busy day, and I was covering an extra list because a colleague was unwell. I was just about coping but I was tired, and I hadn't even had time to go to the toilet. One of the receptionists came to ask me to see 'just one more' patient who had been booked in error with another nurse who is away on holiday. I was just about to call the patient in, when our healthcare assistant came into my room and started talking to me about how stressed he was feeling. I wanted to be supportive, but I just didn't have the energy to give him much attention. I just carried on with my paperwork and didn't really make eye contact, and then said, 'I have to see a patient now….' As he left my room, I felt really guilty that I hadn't been as supportive as I wanted to be. I had hit overload! At home that evening I could not stop thinking about my colleague and how I had not listened when he asked me to, so I ended up feeling miserable all evening and couldn't get to sleep with my busy mind."*

Let's think a bit more about the example of Yasmine and explore her possible values and needs:

Values: What might be some of Yasmine's long-term values?	Professionalism, connection, teamwork, balance, care, compassion
Needs: What might have been some of her short-term needs that arose in this moment and in this situation?	There were several important physical needs including food, water and rest. She had needs relating to effectiveness and managing her time well, as well as connection and support for her colleague
Actions and strategies: What choices could Yasmine make to help meet her needs? What actions could she choose that are in line with her values? Brainstorm as many solutions as possible…	• Take a short comfort break for food and drink • Go for a walk to re-energise and get more focus and clarity before seeing the next patient • Set boundaries about extra workload • Explain to her colleague that she cares how he is feeling but it's hard to focus when she is so busy. Ask if he could postpone the conversation until tomorrow • Talk to a colleague or ask for help if she is feeling overwhelmed • What else could she try…?

PAUSE AND REFLECT: Values, needs and actions

Now it's time to reflect on your own example. Can you think of a recent time when you struggled to meet some of your own needs, or drifted away from following your inner **Guide**? This might be a situation at home or at work. Make a note of it here:

Example: Choose a situation where you struggled to meet your needs or follow your inner **Guide**.	
Values: What are the long-term values that are relevant to you in this situation? What's most important?	
Needs: What were the important short-term needs that arose at this moment and in this situation?	
Actions and strategies: What choices could you make to help meet some of these needs? What actions could you choose that are in line with your values? Brainstorm as many solutions as possible…	

When you don't meet your needs

When you are not making time for your own needs and self-care, it can be difficult to show up as the person you truly want to be at work. Our days are full, fast and frantic, and if you are not getting enough rest, regular meals or time to relax, it's difficult to respond effectively to the complex needs of patients or colleagues. If you are not feeling heard, understood or supported yourself, you may feel overwhelmed at the challenges of listening to and caring for your patients.

The emotional toll of letting your energy tanks run dry, and running on empty, is huge. It will have an impact on you – leading to exhaustion, low mood, anxiety and burnout – and on those around you – as feelings of resentment, guilt and helplessness start to affect your responses and behaviour at home and at work.

So, before you hit crisis point, it's essential that you learn to recognise the early warning signs. Why not try to **NAME** your value or need before you find yourself running on empty?

EXERCISE: NAME your values and needs

Notice your value or need: pause and become aware that one of your needs has not been met or that you are moving away from a core value in some way.

Allow yourself space to pause and ground yourself in the present moment, using your five senses to notice what you can see, hear, touch, smell and taste.

Ask yourself what *Matters* most. Which are the most important needs that you would like to focus on in this situation? What wider values are important to you?

Engage in a valued activity – choose an action that follows your **Guide** and do this with your full attention.

Finding ways to meet your needs

Having a clear understanding of your values and needs allows you to start to take responsibility for meeting them in a more consistent and healthy way. You can also develop greater compassion for yourself in the times that your needs are not fully met.

You can choose multiple different strategies to meet a particular need. For example, you could meet a need for connection by seeing friends, playing with a family pet, connecting via social media, or singing with a local choir. It's important to keep your strategies fluid and flexible and adapt them to each situation.

We will focus more on planning flexible goals and actions to meet your needs in *Chapter 2*.

Anna, Practice Pharmacist: *"I'm so busy with all the different jobs I have to get done in the day, it's hard to prioritise or work out what to do next. I get really bogged down with all my work tasks, so I constantly leave late and then I have arguments with my partner because we hardly spend any time together in the evenings."*

Anna is feeling overloaded by all her different jobs and priorities. She decides to use the **NAME** steps to work through all the different needs that she's trying to juggle. One day as she drives home from work, rather than rushing straight into her evening, she takes five minutes to pause and reflect on her needs:

Notice: she begins by taking a slow breath and becoming aware of all her different needs at that moment: *"There's a lot going on for me when I come home from work..."*

Allow: Anna grounds herself in the present moment by pausing and noticing three sounds in the background, then she gently stretches her arms and shoulders and takes a few slow breaths.

What *Matters*? *"At this moment, at the end of the day, I feel hungry, tired and drained. I have a need for **rest** and **relaxation** and **sustenance.** I'm also really wanting **connection** with my partner, but I can notice that I'm also quite uptight and need some **space** to wind down before I'll have the energy to fully connect."*

Engage in a valued activity: I'm going to go for a 10 minute walk before I go in the house and use the time to help me transition from my busy working day. I will also have a fruit tea. Tomorrow I might try doing 10 minutes of yoga and see which is most helpful. Later tonight I will ask my partner to cook dinner with me, so we have some quality time together.

1.5 Purpose and meaning

Finding meaning and purpose can be helpful when we are feeling uncertain or lost. This can help us to make decisions and choices about the direction of our lives and find ways to use our limited time and energy in ways that feel purposeful and meaningful.

Many people often wish to be 'happy', yet excessive striving for happiness can leave us feeling stressed, frustrated and anxious. We risk focusing too much on ourselves, trying to satisfy our wants and needs, and measuring ourselves and our success against other people, so we invariably come up short.

In contrast, seeking purpose and meaning often involves looking outwards, finding ways to make a difference in the world and participating in things that are bigger than we are. And through our contribution to the wider community, we may find greater fulfilment, satisfaction and contentment, develop improved optimism, and become better able to cope with setbacks.

PAUSE AND REFLECT: What's your purpose for working?

Work can provide purpose and meaning and also fulfils many needs. It also provides the ability to sustain a lifestyle we choose, support ourselves and our loved ones, and allows us to use our skills, strengths and training to maximise our potential.

Look at the following social media post by a junior doctor who is seeking advice about their future career choice. There are several answers from GPs as to why they have chosen this career.

Think about which values might relate to each answer, and what might give each individual a sense of meaning and purpose. We have made some suggestions for the first few answers – try adding your own thoughts to complete the table:

Tobias, Junior Doctor: *"I'm starting GP training in August but I'm beginning to wonder if I have made the right choice and whether it's the best career option for me. So, help, please! What are the reasons that you chose GP as a career? What keeps you going to work even after a busy or stressful day? Is your work leading to a fulfilling life?"*

Answer	Possible values
I chose to be a GP because I value my family and I want to have a flexible career that allows me to work part-time and fits around my life commitments.	*Flexibility, family*
I really enjoy getting to know my patients over time, seeing them through different illnesses through their life. I also like the variety – having to know a bit about everything, never knowing what's going to present next, is very stimulating and keeps me interested and enthusiastic!	*Relationships, variety, learning*

Working in primary care offers many opportunities to diversify and develop a portfolio career. I've become a GP Trainer, and I have some involvement with local politics and medico-legal work. Many of my colleagues have diverse special interests, including dermatology, palliative care, medical writing, and some are even entrepreneurs.	
I enjoy working with my practice team. I have great relationships with my partners and colleagues and it's their support that gets me through stressful days. No matter how difficult the day is, we always seem to find time for a quick chat and a joke to lift our spirits.	
What is your purpose or meaning at work? What are the reasons that you chose your career? Which values may be involved?	

Purpose, meaning and balance

For many clinicians, a sense of purpose comes from working in a caring professional role, undertaking meaningful and satisfying work that contributes to wider society, and being able to contribute to the wellbeing of patients and colleagues.

A loss of this vital sense of meaning may contribute to problems such as work-related stress and burnout. These may also arise when life is out of balance, and we are not meeting our important needs for wellbeing. We will talk more about this in later chapters.

For now, let's look at some simple examples of ways to find a greater sense of meaning and purpose:

Strategy	Examples	What could you try?
Give and receive support and strengthen relationships	Become an educator, mentor or appraiser Socialise with colleagues outside work Join a committee or a leadership organisation Join a sports club or walking group	

Contribute to your local community and the wider world	Get involved with your local social prescribing team to set up or become part of a Parkrun initiative Give a talk to local schools about your role Do some shopping for an elderly neighbour	
Connect with others, finding ways to share your hopes, fears, successes and failures	Talk through a mistake at work with a supportive colleague or listen to someone else who is struggling Eat your lunch in the coffee room and ask colleagues how their day is going	
Focus outside yourself on causes, pursuits and wider responsibilities	Find ways to make your workplace greener Get involved with national or political organisations	
Pursue professional or educational goals that you find personally meaningful	Seek out training to help you develop new skills and expertise Take a course in something completely different from work	
Keep a balance between your pursuit of pleasure and purpose	Ensure that you include enjoyable family activities in your week Get back to a regular hobby or exercise class	
Find ways to show respect and value others	Ensure you are an equal opportunities workplace Stand up for yourself or someone disadvantaged if you observe discrimination	

1.6 Personal qualities

Acknowledging and developing your personal qualities can also be an important part of living according to your values. Attributes such as patience, kindness, honesty and reliability can move us towards values such as professionalism or connection with others. We may use patience and persistence when working with vulnerable elderly patients or those with learning disabilities, or when supporting a struggling colleague to develop a skill that they find difficult. Our personal qualities will both influence *how* we do things as well as affect our choices in *what* we do, as we follow our inner **Guide**.

PAUSE AND REFLECT: Personal strengths and qualities

- What are some of your personal strengths?
- What are you good at?
- What do you enjoy and care about?
- Are there any ways to appreciate and further develop these qualities?

1.7 Troubleshooting finding your inner Guide

I'm not sure what my values and needs are

Following your **Guide** is an ongoing process, and you may need to revisit your values and needs many times. Try to focus on the two or three most important needs and values that are affecting you right now. Remember to come back to this section on your inner **Guide** regularly to update your values as your interests and priorities develop and evolve over time.

I have so many values – I don't know which to choose!

If you are enthusiastic about multiple values, you might find it hard to narrow them down. That's fine too. Why not try different ones on for size? You could experiment with actions relating to different values and notice the effect on your life. If you are feeling bogged down and restricted by over-focus on values such as responsibility or organisation, why not try exploring different ones such as autonomy and spontaneity? Take yourself on an unexpected shopping spree or go for an unplanned walk somewhere completely new. Notice the impact of trying out this new action.

I'm overwhelmed and unsure how to get started!

It's not necessary to make huge changes, even if the problems that you care about are important issues. Instead, you can start small and plan tiny micro-steps in the direction of your values. We talk more about these in *Chapter 2*. These tiny changes can have a surprising impact in opening up possibilities and developing your confidence to try something new.

I feel alone – no one shares my values

Your values are your own unique perspective on the world, although they may be shaped by your experiences and your culture. However, it can be an isolating and lonely experience to feel alone and that no one understands or shares your most important or personal values.

It may help to actively seek out others who share your values – to find a tribe of people who understand and support your perspective. Finding just one other person who shares a value might be enough, or you may find a whole community to offer encouragement. This could be face-to-face or via an online or virtual group.

My values are conflicting or competing: what should I do?

Values and needs are not the same as specific strategies or actions. You can hold multiple values at once. You might value commitment in relationships, personal autonomy and space, and your sense of security and stability, all at the same time. It is the strategies that we choose, and how much time and energy we choose to put into these different activities, that may sometimes create conflict. Remember, there is no 'correct' or 'perfect' solution – it's usually a question of balance or trying things out to see what happens.

Prioritising and considering your essential needs can also be helpful. Imagine being on a boat that is sinking, and you can only keep a handful of your values or needs, tossing the rest overboard. Which are you left with? Does this help to prioritise your decisions? We look more closely at making helpful choices in *Chapter 4*.

Chapter summary: using your Guide

- Your inner **Guide** acts as a compass, which points in the direction of your most important values and the things in life that matter most to you.

- Following your **Guide** involves asking yourself questions such as: Who and what do I care about? What kind of person do I want to be? What do I want to stand for in my life?

- The next step is to plan 'towards actions' which move you in the direction of an important value, even if these involve overcoming challenges or difficulty.

- To thrive, we must NAME our values and needs and actively respond to them before we hit 'empty':
  - Notice your value or need
  - Allow yourself space to pause and connect with the present moment
  - Ask yourself what Matters most?
  - Engage in a valued activity with your full attention

- Finding ways to increase your sense of meaning and purpose in life can lead to improved fulfilment, contentment and optimism.

Final thoughts

What are the most important messages for you from this chapter?

Take an action step

What are your next steps? What actions will you take as a result of reading this chapter?

Are there any values you are thinking about differently, or needs you are going to prioritise?

02 Ready for Action

> - Are you prepared, proactive and meeting your personal and professional goals, or are you overwhelmed and often procrastinating over decisions or plans?
>
> - Do you feel in control of your daily actions and routines, or are you floundering under an ever-growing list of tasks and daily responsibilities?
>
> - Do you worry about whether you will achieve things to a high enough standard, so you push yourself relentlessly or avoid doing it altogether?
>
> - Do you want to find the motivation to achieve what matters most whilst acknowledging your own needs and interests? Keep reading …

2.1 The importance of taking action

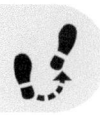

Taking action involves doing what matters, even when facing stress, difficulties, emotional changes and challenging events. It's often easier to change our actions than our attitudes or emotions. Trying out new ways of behaving, or consciously reacting to things differently, can create an opportunity for positive change.

Taking action involves making choices and balancing how much time and energy we put into different types of activity. In *Chapter 1*, we met our inner **Guide**, becoming motivated by what we value and care about, and recognising our important needs. The next step is to get **Ready for Action** and find concrete ways to live out these values. This involves:

- Doing things because they are important or meaningful, even if we also experience negative thoughts, difficult feelings or lack of motivation

- Being willing to try something new rather than staying stuck in old habits or patterns of behaviour

- Planning realistic changes which help us move towards our values in tiny achievable steps.

Misha, newly qualified GP: *"I'm spending all my time at work and as it's so busy, I can't seem to fit anything else in. My team are great – but I keep thinking that I'm not doing as well as everyone else and worrying that I'm letting myself down. I'm constantly stressed and anxious and I can't remember when I last enjoyed being at work. I keep trying to remind myself why I went through my training and all the effort it took to get here, but every morning I just want to hide under the duvet and stay at home. I'd love to get back to feeling more positive and motivated."*

Misha qualified as a GP about 6 months ago and has found the transition from being a GP Registrar very hard. She feels anxious and overwhelmed at work, despite having a supportive team around her. Misha is starting to feel quite low and demoralised, and her concentration and efficiency at work are starting to suffer. Recently she became very tearful after a long and busy day as duty doctor and is starting to wonder whether she would be better off giving up working as a GP altogether.

Misha may benefit from engaging with her inner **Guide** to help her start to plan some simple Towards actions that keep moving her towards her values and also meet some of her important needs. As we progress through this chapter, we will explore how she might go about this.

2.2 What is taking action?

Actions are how we can influence the world around us through our behaviour. When we carry out actions that are congruent with and support our values, we are more likely to feel fulfilled and that life has meaning and purpose.

So, if your value is teamwork, you might take action by ensuring that you make time in your week to have meaningful discussions with colleagues. Alternatively, if you value connection with your family, you might ensure that you make space for family time at weekends and have a meal together in the evening without distractions. Taking action does not have to be a major life change but may involve making small tweaks to your routine which change the quality of your activities and interactions and bring you closer to your values.

Actions can also have an impact on your mood and stress levels. Spending time with a close friend may lift your mood and make you feel upbeat and positive. Alternatively, avoiding social interaction can make you feel isolated, low and more prone to worry.

External and internal actions

External actions take place in the physical world and can be observed by other people, such as what we do or say. As you arrive at work each day, you may carry out many actions including turning on your computer, making yourself a coffee or chatting to a colleague. We can also consider *not* doing something as a type of action. Not doing something could be helpful, or it could involve procrastination – putting off important tasks and instead getting stuck in social media or watching TV.

There are also *internal* actions, which take place within our mind and cannot necessarily be seen by other people. These usually involve thinking about something repeatedly, such as getting caught up in worries, doubt, mentally planning for the future, or repetitive self-critical thoughts and recriminations.

Other people may not be able to observe the thoughts that arise during internal actions, but their impact can often be seen in the outer world. When you are actively listening to and interacting with a colleague, it is usually obvious that you are present and engaged in the conversation. But if you are caught up in worries about what you are going to do with your next patient, you may appear preoccupied or distant, stare into space, hesitate when answering, or you may even seem uninterested in what your colleague is saying.

We will look in more detail at how to cope with intrusive thoughts and worry in future chapters. For now, we will focus on making active choices about our visible, external actions. And, as we focus on taking steps towards what matters most to us, *in spite* of what is going on internally, this can also help to manage mental preoccupation.

PAUSE AND REFLECT: Bring a memory to mind

Take a moment to think about a recent time in which you felt a sense of pleasure or enjoyment, or that life was fulfilling and meaningful. It often helps to pick something small or simple, such as sharing a joke or a drink with friends or colleagues, a time on holiday when you saw a wonderful view, or a moment when you felt fully engaged in an activity such as playing sport. Try to bring this memory to mind in detail, using all your senses. Now answer the following questions about the memory that you have chosen:

Where are you? Take a moment to notice your surroundings including the colours, sounds, smells and sensations	
What are you doing? Describe your actions in detail	

How engaged or present are you in this activity? Are you giving it your full attention or is your mind elsewhere?	
What emotions can you notice? Are there feelings such as joy, happiness or contentment? Do any other feelings arise, such as sadness, regret or sorrow, as you focus on this memory?	
How are you treating yourself, others and the world around you? What personal qualities are you demonstrating?	
What can you learn from this? What actions, behaviours or personal qualities would you like to bring to your daily life?	

Here are the responses from Misha, the newly qualified GP who is feeling overwhelmed at work:

Where are you? Take a moment to notice your surroundings including the colours, sounds, smells, and sensations	I'm lying on a sunbed on holiday in Portugal. I can see the blue pool next to me, and it's a lovely sunny day. It's very peaceful and there are beautiful purple flowers around the pool. I can see my partner next to me.
What are you doing? Describe your actions in detail	I'm reading my book and have just looked up to take in the view.
How engaged or present are you in this activity? Are you giving it your full attention or is your mind elsewhere?	I feel really engaged in this moment. I'm not thinking about work at all! I am just enjoying my book and the surroundings.
What emotions can you notice? Are there feelings such as joy, happiness or contentment? Do any other feelings arise, such as sadness, regret or sorrow, as you focus on this memory?	At the time I felt really happy, content and peaceful. Now I'm looking back, I can remember those feelings, and I also feel sad that life is so difficult at the moment.

How are you treating yourself, others and the world around you? What personal qualities are you demonstrating?	I'm being very open and friendly to my partner and to everyone around me. I'm also treating myself with kindness and giving myself permission to relax and enjoy the holiday.
What can you learn from this? What actions, behaviours or personal qualities would you like to bring to your daily life?	I'd like to bring more relaxation and enjoyment into my life at the moment. This was such a lovely moment – it feels really far away from how I'm living right now.

2.3 From values to actions

Our values are like the roots of a tree. They provide the support, strength, stability and nourishment that enable the tree to grow strong and healthy. The earth and the ground that the roots sit in will also affect the growth of the tree. This is our environment, our background, and the life events that all affect our attitudes and beliefs.

From our values come our goals and plans for the future. These are the branches of the tree stretching upwards and outwards in many different directions. They might include smaller twigs, such as plans for the next day or week, as well as larger branches which represent long-term plans for the next months or even years.

Finally, we have individual tiny actions that create the overall shape and beauty of the tree. These are the hundreds or even thousands of leaves, which all together provide the tree with energy to develop and grow. Your values, goals and actions work together to enable you to thrive, influenced by your background and environment.

Actions and habits

Our choices of actions often follow repeated patterns or habits. Habitual behaviours may feel comfortable and familiar – like a well-worn pair of slippers that are past their best but are difficult to part with. Although you may know that the actions you sometimes take are not in your best interests, you might get stuck in the habit of working long hours or at weekends to keep up, skipping breaks, or disconnecting from colleagues. You continue these habitual actions because they have become your way of coping, even though they may be unhelpful and clash with other important values and needs, such as self-care and being a nurturing parent or supportive friend.

The good news is that we don't have to stick with old habits if they are no longer working. We can choose our actions and we can use this to take control of the direction of our lives.

The first step is to take some time to pay attention and notice your habitual actions. Ask yourself whether a particular activity or habit is adding something positive to your life – is it enjoyable, important or uplifting in some way? Or is it acting as a 'life-drain' – sucking up your time and making you feel more negative, low, or lacking in energy or confidence?

Life-boosting actions:

- Are enjoyable and uplifting
- Are important or meaningful
- Offer a sense of achievement or satisfaction

Life-draining actions:

- Lower your mood or energy
- Don't add value to your life
- Involve avoiding or putting off things that are important

PAUSE AND REFLECT: Noticing your daily actions

Think about the past week and what you did on a typical working day and another day when you had free time. Make a list of what you did on each day and include as many actions as you can. Try to include small things, such as taking a shower or making a drink, as well as longer activities, such as meeting with colleagues, going out to meet a friend for dinner or doing household chores.

How long did each action or activity last for? Then decide, on balance, whether it was life-boosting or life-draining. The aim is to discover any actions, however seemingly insignificant, like greeting the shopkeeper or stopping mid-morning for a cup of tea, which made a difference to your day.

A working day: make a list of actions during the day	How long did you do it for?	Was it life-boosting (B) or life-draining (D)?

A day with free time: make a list of actions during the day	How long did you do it for?	Was it life-boosting (B) or life-draining (D)?

PAUSE AND REFLECT: Noticing your actions

Now go back to the list of activities and actions that you spend your time on. Ask yourself:

- **Is this a TOWARDS action** that moves you in the direction of your values and needs and following your inner **Guide**? Underline or highlight all the Towards actions and things you are doing which are a good 'fit' with who you want to be.

- **Where are the clashes?** What are you doing that creates conflict with your values or needs, or causes you concern or distress? Underline or highlight some of the **AWAY actions** in a different colour.

- **Notice the differences:** Are there any actions which had a variable quality to them that made them life-draining or life-boosting on different occasions? What made the difference? Was it *how* you completed the action, your *attitude* towards it or the *amount of time* you spent on it?

Write what you have discovered from this exercise here:

2.4 Are you living according to your values?

Most health professionals are highly skilled at setting goals, meeting targets, and planning how to cope with possible difficulties. But it may also be important to set aside the space and time to actively apply what you already know in your daily life. It's also important to avoid being rigid and ensure that your plans and goals remain balanced, flexible and adaptable to changing circumstances.

You can start by making small changes to bring your life more in line with your values. What would life look like if you were meeting your important needs and living according to your values? What limits you or gets in the way of this?

Take a look at the following diagram and think about how close you are to 'hitting the target' in different areas of your life. We have suggested some life areas that are important to many people, and you can add any other important areas, such as spirituality, or specific relationships, such as being a parent.

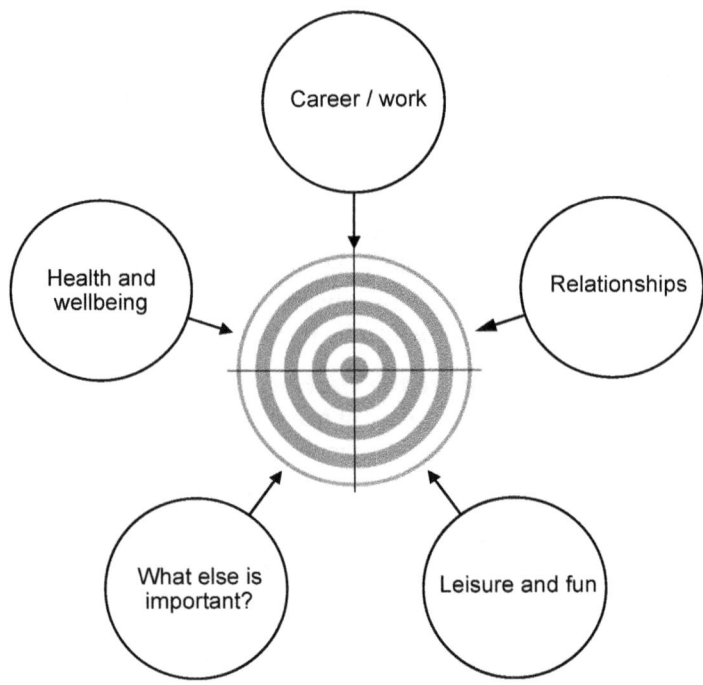

We asked Misha, the newly qualified GP who is feeling overwhelmed by her work, to complete this exercise. Here is her 'target' diagram:

"This was an interesting exercise to carry out. I'm not really 'hitting the bullseye' in any of my life areas at the moment, but some are further out than others. Work is probably the closest in, as I'm going every day and putting in a lot of effort, but I'm not enjoying myself. Relationships are much further out – I keep arguing with my partner as I'm irritable when I get home, and I hardly have time to see my friends or family! I'm not unhealthy – I eat fairly well and look after myself – but I don't get round to exercise at the moment. For leisure, I mainly watch TV or play on my phone, but often I'm not paying attention and not really enjoying myself. What else is important? I love my cat and he is really well looked after!"

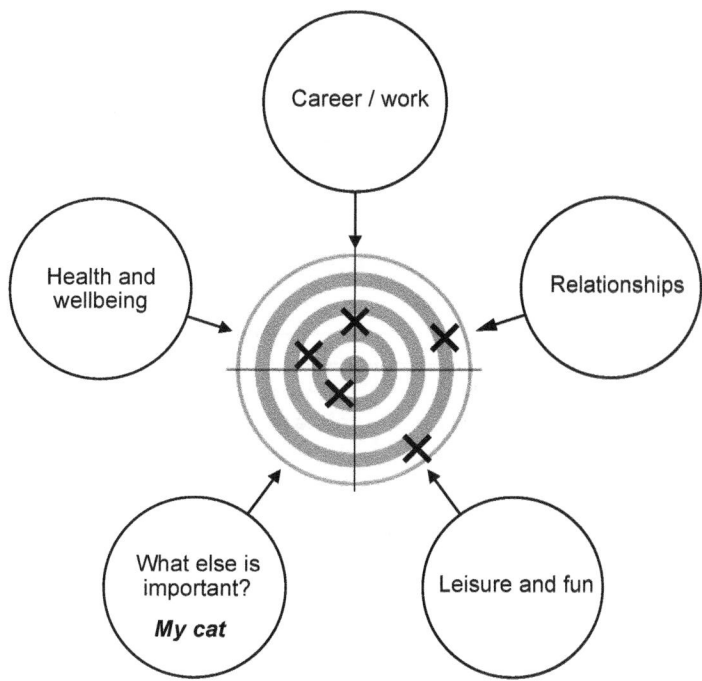

2.5 Plans, goals and actions

The next step is to start making plans, setting goals and scheduling specific actions:

- **Plans** involve deciding what is most important in the long term.

- **Goals** involve thinking about what we would like to achieve in the short or medium term.

- **Actions** are small, specific, concrete and immediate steps towards a goal or a long-term plan.

Micro-actions

Micro-actions are tiny actions that only take a short time to complete, ideally between 2 and 10 minutes. Most of us are incredibly busy, with many tasks that are non-flexible, and may have little room for making major changes in our activity patterns.

Carrying out a micro-action is unlikely to completely resolve a major life problem, but it is a step in the right direction. It also helps us to become less rigid or stuck in negative habits of thinking and behaviour, increasing our psychological and behavioural flexibility.

TAKE ACTION

Take a few minutes to complete the following table. Can you commit to at least one micro-action that you are confident you can complete within the next few days?

Pick a value or a life domain that is important to you	List some activities that relate to this value	Pick one activity and break it into smaller steps. Can you plan a micro-action?

Here is Misha's completed chart:

Pick a value or a life domain that is important to you	List some activities that relate to this value	Pick one activity and break it into smaller steps. Can you plan a micro-action?
Relaxation and enjoyment	Playing my flute Reading Relaxing more at home	Spend 10 minutes looking for local music groups Ask my friend to recommend an enjoyable book Have a bubble bath or paint my toenails
Relationships – partner and friends	Spend quality time with my partner Make time to see my friends and family	Book a trip to the cinema for next weekend with my partner Print one of my wedding photos to take to work Send a text to my friend Daniella Phone my sister
Physical activity	Try to regularly do some physical activity to wind down and destress	Go for a short walk at lunchtime to stretch my legs and get out of the surgery Ask my neighbour to go for a walk at the weekend Look for times of Zumba classes at the leisure centre

Let's get specific...

Now pick one to three activities from the list above. It's helpful to write them down, which gives an increased sense of commitment that can help you get them done. For each action, ask yourself:

- What am I going to do?

- Why is this important? What value or need is it linked to?

- Where and when will I do it?

- Who will I do it with?

- How often will I do it, and how long will I do it for?

Finish by asking yourself: How confident am I? How likely is it that I will do this (on a scale of 1–10)?

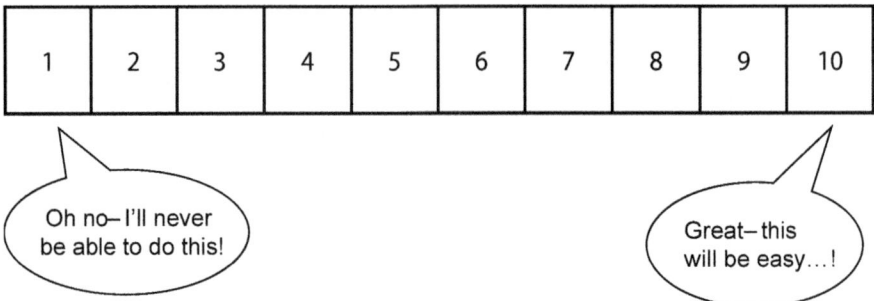

1	2	3	4	5	6	7	8	9	10

Oh no— I'll never be able to do this!

Great— this will be easy…!

Aim for a confidence or likelihood level of **8, 9 or 10** that you will carry out this action. If your score is lower, you may need to make your planned action more achievable or realistic. Think: What would make this easier to carry out? Can I make it into a smaller step? Can I ask someone for help or support?

For each action complete the following table:

What am I going to do?	
Why is this important? What value or need is it linked to?	
Where and when will I do it?	
Who will I do it with?	
How often will I do it? How long will I do it for?	
How likely is it that I will do this (1–10)? Aim for a score of 8, 9 or 10!	
What might get in the way of doing this? How could I make it easier to carry out? Can I make it smaller or shorter, or ask for support?	

Here is Misha's completed chart:

What am I going to do?	I will go for a walk at lunchtime when I'm at work
Why is this important? What value or need is it linked to?	I really need to get a break and get outside during the working day. This will help me to recharge and might make me more efficient in the afternoon
Where and when will I do it?	I will go after I finish my morning surgery and tasks
Who will I do it with?	I could ask one of my colleagues to come with me so we can have a chat and a catch-up
How often will I do it? How long will I do it for?	I will aim to do this at least twice a week for 10 minutes
How likely is it that I will do this (1–10)? Aim for a score of 8, 9 or 10!	Around 6 or 7/10
What might get in the way of doing this? How could I make it easier to carry out? Can I make it smaller or shorter, or ask for support?	I might be busy and forget or feel too tired to go. I might have so much work to get through that I stay in front of my computer through lunchtime To make it easier, I will plan a shorter time, just 5 minutes. I will remind myself that this is important and might help me concentrate on work afterwards

Notice what happened

After trying any new action, it's helpful to take a few minutes to think about what happened. Ask yourself:

What had I planned to do? What did I try?	
Was this action linked to any of my important values?	
What were the short-term effects of doing this?	
What might be the long-term effects?	
What can I learn from this?	
How can I build on this? What will I try next (different or the same)?	

If the action didn't quite go according to plan, there are some other helpful questions:

What got in the way? e.g.: I ran out of time, I forgot, it was too difficult or something else important came up…	
Is this still important? If not, what else could I try?	
What could make it easier next time? Do I need to break it into smaller steps or change my expectations in some way?	
How can I remind myself to do it?	

Here's what happened when Misha tried her action out:

"I had planned to go for a walk for 10 minutes at least twice a week at lunchtime. I only went once but I walked for 15 minutes which was longer than I planned. Taking time out of the day probably made me more productive and I enjoyed it as well. It linked to the value of taking care of myself and made me more relaxed. It's worth the effort! On one of the days, I had an unexpected extra patient, so it was harder to get away, but I will try to go on both days that I planned to next week. I think it is very important and not too difficult for me to fit in. I could aim to go for a shorter time – perhaps just 5 minutes walking around the car park would make a difference. I will set an alarm on my phone to remind me to go."

2.6 What gets in the way?

Even though we may have the best intentions, it can sometimes be hard to carry out actions that take us towards our values. When faced with challenging situations, we may get caught up in distressing thoughts, emotions and body sensations and experience a strong urge to try to reduce this discomfort. However, this often leads to choosing 'Away actions' which move us away from our values and the direction our inner **Guide** is pointing.

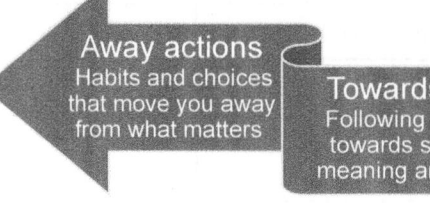

Away actions usually involve trying to reduce difficult feelings or distress. However, in the long term, these often move us away from the people and things that matter most. **Towards actions** are in line with our values and fit with who we want to be, and usually lead to a greater sense of satisfaction, enjoyment and control over life.

Abdul, Practice Pharmacist:
Abdul wants to do more exercise to improve his fitness and lose weight, but he finds it hard to motivate himself after work. He spends most evenings slumped in his chair dozing or watching TV. Being sedentary in front of the TV is an Away action which moves him away from his values of physical activity, health and self-care. But he makes this choice because of his feelings of fatigue, and negative thoughts saying, "I'll just look ridiculous and weak if I go to the gym, I haven't been for years, and I won't be as fit as all the other guys."

Bernice, Practice Nurse:
Bernice has been a nurse for many years and would really like to develop some new skills and apply to train as a nurse practitioner. But she feels so anxious about submitting her application that she procrastinates and misses the deadline. This is also an Away action, driven by feelings of anxiety and fear, and negative thoughts about being "found out" and "not being up to the job". These have got in the way of moving towards her values of self-development and career satisfaction.

Action spoilers

Action spoilers are examples of some common types of Away actions. These may involve physical sensations, emotions, thoughts or actions. Take a look at the list below. Do you recognise any action spoilers that frequently get in the way of achieving important goals?

Action spoiler: common types of Away actions		Do you recognise this?	What do you notice? How does it affect you?
Emotions	Negative feelings such as anxiety, fear, sadness, anger, guilt or shame		

Physical sensations	Body sensations such as fatigue, lethargy, heaviness, pain and tightness		
Thoughts and beliefs	Negative thoughts and predictions about what might go wrong		
	Underestimating or doubting your ability or performance		
	Being too demanding, with excessively high expectations and unrealistic goals		
	Focusing on short-term discomfort and ignoring the long-term benefits of change		
	Criticising or judging your own performance		
Behaviour	Delay tactics, procrastination or avoidance		
	Waiting until you feel like doing something before getting started		
	Not asking for help or taking on too much responsibility		
	Trying to complete too much at once or underestimating the time required		
	Not being assertive or expressing your own opinion or needs to others		
	Spending time with people or in places that make it harder to stick to your goals		
	Avoiding new challenges and staying in your comfort zone		

Think of one or more times that you wanted to do something but didn't get round to doing it. What got in the way? What examples of action spoilers and Away actions can you notice in yourself?

2.7 Take a Towards step

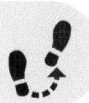

To achieve our important goals, we may sometimes need to take a Towards action even when this might involve some discomfort, or when various action spoilers pop up and try to get in the way. Before we deliver a presentation to a large audience, perhaps we can accept that we may feel a little nervous beforehand. Or we might choose to study for an important exam, even when tempted to go out for drinks with friends.

We can carry out a Towards action which moves us towards something important, even in the presence of uncomfortable thoughts and feelings. This may not be easy! We will learn more skills in how to do this as we progress through the book.

Think back to the action spoilers that you identified in the previous exercise, which have got in the way and stopped you from doing something that you wanted to achieve. Can you plan a micro-action, that moves you towards one of your values?

To make this action step small and achievable, you may need to let go of unrealistic goals and focus on making progress in the direction of a long-term plan rather than making the whole step in one leap. You may also need to seek support or help from others and be flexible in how you approach your goals.

Try to plan two or three Towards action steps that might help you move past your action spoilers. Can you commit to trying these in the near future?

Stepping outside your comfort zone

Being **Ready for Action** also involves stepping outside our comfort zone as we explore new ways of living and discover how different actions can bring our values to life. This involves accepting uncertainty – we need to be willing to try something different, even when we are not sure exactly what will happen. This can be uncomfortable at first, because old habits often feel safe and secure, even if they are not very healthy or positive. But like all great adventures, it can also lead you in all kinds of new and exciting directions.

It can be helpful to pause and reflect when you notice this discomfort:

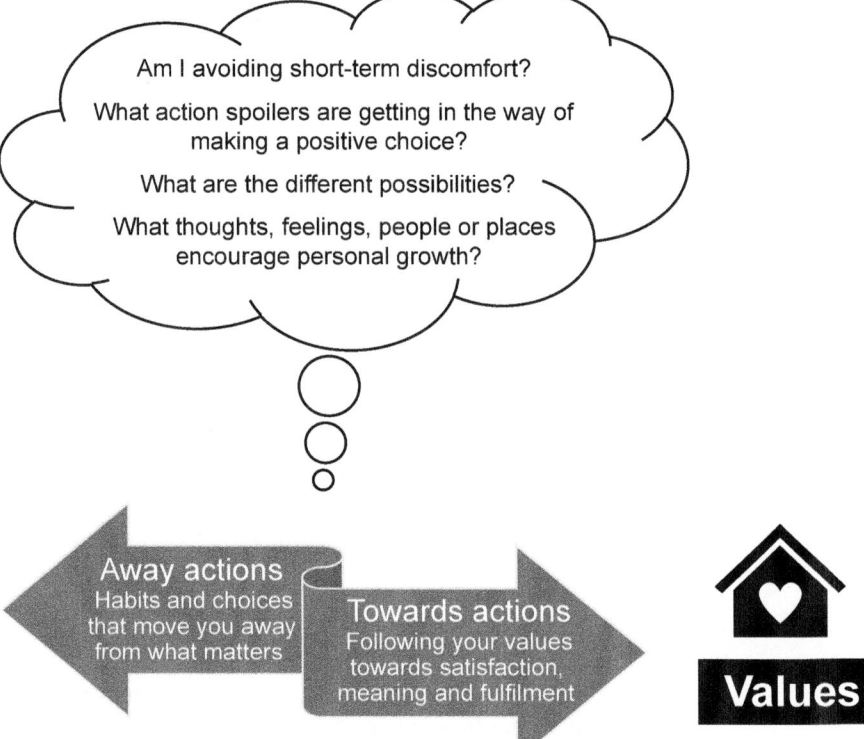

Ready to take action: myths and facts

Myth	Fact	Towards action
I have to be motivated and in the right mood before I can get started	We can generate motivation by trying something and gradually build momentum from the positive feedback of getting started.	✔ Behave as if you feel more motivated or enthusiastic and the feeling will catch up ✔ Take one small step to get started ✔ Experiment and see what happens
I'm too tired or lethargic to start. I need to rest and save my energy	You can often energise yourself through gradually increasing activity levels. Over time, your physical and mental energy will grow as you become stronger and fitter.	✔ Break the task into smaller steps ✔ Start low, go slow, and build up gradually ✔ Allow feelings of energy and achievement to slowly catch up
There isn't enough time to get the important things done	Prioritise and make sure that you get through the most important tasks first. You might also need to set boundaries around your time, especially for work tasks which may feel never-ending.	✔ Think: what is essential to achieve today? ✔ Do priority tasks first, even if they are the least enjoyable ✔ Be realistic: plan small, achievable actions rather than attempting too much ✔ Stop before you are exhausted or hit 'empty'
I find it hard to get started with tasks that I don't enjoy or find difficult, even if they are important	Some important tasks are not very enjoyable, such as completing a tax return or preparing for an appraisal. You may need to take a breath, choose to accept some short-term discomfort, and take a micro-step to get started.	✔ Think about your values: is it important for you or someone you care about? ✔ What are the negative consequences of avoiding the task? ✔ Visualise how satisfied you will feel when it's completed ✔ Enlist help: share the load or find a task buddy or supporter ✔ Plan a micro-action: I will do 10 minutes preparation and then take a break
The things I want are impossible; there's no point even trying to achieve them	If something's important it may be worth putting in some extra effort. Or do you need to adjust your goals and make them more achievable? Just take a tiny step – don't expect a giant leap!	✔ Adjust your goals if necessary ✔ Up-skill yourself or ask for help ✔ Get prepared – have the right tools and equipment ready ✔ Keep practising and acknowledge your efforts

PAUSE AND REFLECT: Actions – myths and facts

Have any of the above 'myths' stopped you from trying something?

Which of the Towards action remedies can you try?

2.8 Planning for the long term

Now it's time to dream a little and make some long-term plans, knowing that they are flexible and can be adapted to changing circumstances in the future:

Imagine you are sailing towards your dream destination. You are heading towards a beautiful island which is due north, but the wind is against you. In order to get there, you adjust your sails to the wind and tack north-west and then north-east diagonally, heading in a general northerly direction. En route, you encounter a storm and take shelter on an island to stay safe and then discover that you actually prefer this island to the one you were aiming for. This demonstrates how we can be flexible and adapt our goals and aspirations according to our needs and values and the context. Like sailing, life is about enjoying the journey and not simply reaching the destination.

Making life plans

What would life look like if you were 'living the dream' and hitting the target in all areas of your life – acting in line with your values, meeting important needs and being in places and with people you care about? What would you be **DOING** differently or doing more of?

Spend a moment writing down your ideal, aspirational, even if somewhat unrealistic, dream life here:

Now we are going make this a little more concrete and realistic. You may have to let go of things which are completely out of reach, but you can include important long-term plans or directions of travel. Pick one or two life areas that you would most like to work on, that would make a meaningful impact to your life.

EXERCISE: Making life plans and setting goals

Chose a life area   Work

What are your long-term plans or aspirations?	What are your most important values and needs relating to this?	What are some short- or medium-term goals that you could aim for?
Take on a management role or develop a specialist interest Retire at 60	Leadership Learning Financial security	Find a training course that would help me develop new skills and knowledge Book a meeting with a financial adviser to discuss retirement planning

Choose a life area:

What are your long-term plans or aspirations?	What are your most important values and needs relating to this?	What are some short- or medium-term goals that you could aim for?

Chapter summary: Ready for Action

- Actions have a powerful influence over how we think and feel.

- Actions are more likely to be enjoyable and life-boosting if they move us towards our values and the person we want to be.

- Choosing specific, relevant and achievable goals can help motivate us to make important changes.

- Making positive choices and completing regular actions can lead to longer-term gains and help us break free from unhelpful patterns.

- Now…. pick an action and try it out. This chapter is about taking action and not just talking about it… follow your inner **Guide** as you get **Ready for Action**!

Final thoughts

What are the most important messages for you from this chapter?

Take an action step

What are your next steps? What actions will you take as a result of reading this chapter?

Are there any regular actions or patterns of behaviour that you might try to practise or develop?

03 Open and Observe

- Are you able to focus on what's most important, or do negative thoughts, worries or distressing memories make it hard to concentrate and get things done?

- Are you able to enjoy the moment, or do feelings of stress and strong emotions affect how you function day to day or interfere with enjoyment and relaxation?

- Do you try hard to rid yourself of difficult thoughts and feelings?

- Are you just too busy to stop and be mindful? Keep reading…

3.1 Open and Observe skills

Learning to **Open and Observe** involves becoming more aware of what's going on inside us, and in the world around. Being able to notice and acknowledge our own thoughts and feelings can help us to understand ourselves, and to step back, make decisions, and cope more effectively under pressure.

In this chapter, we will look at ways to develop skills in learning to **Open and Observe** which include:

- Noticing what's happening in your body and mind, and in the environment around you.

- Recognising your thoughts and feelings without judging them or getting caught up, reacting to them, or wrestling with them.

- Creating space to enable you to choose actions that follow your inner **Guide**, even when difficult thoughts and feelings are present.

3.2 Observe this moment: notice the 'NOW'

Meilin, Practice Nurse: *"I sometimes get so caught up in thinking about work that I can drive all the way home and I have no idea how I got there! Or I might just walk straight past one of my colleagues without saying good morning because I'm worrying about my first patient or what time I will get home that night…"*

How often do you slip into 'automatic pilot' where you are not fully paying attention or aware of what you are doing? At times, this can be helpful, as it frees our mind to drift elsewhere when we don't need to concentrate on routine tasks that we have done many times before. But if it becomes a frequent habit, we may not be really 'present', moment by moment, for much of our lives.

When operating on automatic pilot, we are less able to make active decisions about the best way to cope in a challenging situation. We may be more likely to use old habits of thinking and behaving, which may be unhelpful in the current circumstances.

One of the first skills of **Open and Observe** involves learning to **pause** and **notice** when we have gone into automatic pilot. This increased awareness offers greater choice about how we wish to respond to life's challenges, and can prevent us from falling into the same old mental ruts or habits which may have caused problems in the past. It also gives more opportunity to notice and appreciate the positive moments in life.

EXERCISE: Notice your hands
Hold your hands out with your palms touching. Now slowly start to move your hands and fingers. Notice the sensations in your fingertips, palms and hands, as you gently rub them together for 15–30 seconds.

You have just completed a few seconds of mindfulness!

PAUSE AND REFLECT: Noticing your hands

- What did you notice? What physical sensations were you aware of?

- Did any thoughts pop up in your mind? How about feelings and emotions?

Meilin could try taking a few moments during each day to pause and take a breath or rub her hands together for a few seconds, just to be a little more present and aware. She could also take a few breaths before she gets into the car to drive home. Whilst driving, she can ground herself by noticing the physical sensations of holding the steering wheel, feeling the pressure of her back against the seat, and observing details of the road and traffic around her. Once she arrives home, she might stretch her arms and back, becoming aware of the physical sensations of her body, helping her to transition from work to home.

3.3 Finding flow

In a state of 'flow', we are totally absorbed and deeply focused on a task or activity. Our concentration and focus are heightened, and we do not get caught up by distractions. We let go of our thoughts, worries and plans for the future, as we focus on the here and now. Time flies by as we forget about everything but what we are doing at this moment.

Finding flow usually brings feelings of contentment and satisfaction in whatever we are doing. Have you ever felt fully absorbed by a great book with an exciting storyline? Have you felt 'in the zone' as you played a sport, where time seemed to slow down, and you felt completely connected to and absorbed by the activity? Or had so much fun with a group of friends that the time just flew by? Have you been transfixed by a beautiful sunrise or by a piece of entrancing music that completely captures your attention? These all represent a moment of flow.

We can also experience flow at work, when we are fully engaged in what we are doing and find a sense of satisfaction from completing tasks as we progress through the day.

EXERCISE: Noticing autopilot and flow

Can you think of a time that you were in autopilot, when your mind was so caught up that you didn't notice something else? What were you doing? What were the problems or advantages of being on autopilot in this situation?

How about finding flow? Can you think of any times that you were really engaged in an activity? What helped you to stay focused? How did it feel to be 'in the zone'?

Seeking out flow

It's often easier to find flow when carrying out activities that we find naturally engaging and absorbing. What activities draw you in and hold your interest or attention? It could involve creating art, researching a topic that interests you, playing a sport, or even doing a chore that you find calming or soothing.

Choose an activity and try bringing your full attention to it for just a few minutes. This might help create a sense of flow as you become absorbed without thinking about distractions. If you find this tricky, it's possible to build your skills in focus and attention with only a few minutes of regular practice. One way of doing this is to use your senses, focusing on what you can see, feel, hear and smell, as you carry out the activity. You can describe or name what you sense in your mind to fully bring it to your attention.

3.4 Flexible attention

Callum, GP Partner: *"I don't have problems paying attention. In fact, I get so caught up in what I'm doing that I often don't notice how I'm feeling physically. I often miss lunch or don't drink for ages, because I'm so focused on getting a task completed. And I will keep working until I'm virtually exhausted. My colleagues sometimes say that I don't notice their needs either – in meetings I get so focused on getting the job done that my partners sometimes complain that I haven't listened to their point of view! I just get really focused on one thing and find it hard to see the big picture."*

Shifting your attention

Getting stuck or over-focused on one particular task, viewpoint or mindset is another type of automatic pilot, where we become rigid in our thinking styles or behaviours. Developing **Open and Observe** skills can help us to recognise and step out of these fixed patterns.

If we develop the ability to observe, move and shift our focus, keeping it fluid and flexible, we can avoid getting caught up or 'hooked' by thoughts, or over-focused on a task. This may involve shifting our attention from noticing our environment, moving inwards to acknowledge our inner thoughts and feelings, and then opening back up to our surroundings once more as we decide what to do next.

As we develop flexible attention, we are more able to remain in contact with the present moment, remain aware of our emotions, sensations and thoughts, and continue to act in a way that's helpful in the bigger picture of our lives, following our inner **Guide** and remaining in touch with our values and needs.

EXERCISE: Attention shifting

Use the following exercise to develop your skills in flexible attention, as you shift focus between different aspects of your experience:

- Notice a physical sensation in your body – it may help to exaggerate this by moving your body. Push your feet into the floor, scrunch your toes or stretch your arms up above your head. Pause for 10–20 seconds and notice the physical sensations.

- Now shift your attention to a sound. It might be something you can hear in your environment, or you can create a sound by gently humming or tapping on the desk. Pause for 10–20 seconds in awareness of this sound.

- Shift your attention to something that you can see in your immediate environment. Take 10–20 seconds to really look at this, noticing the object's colours, shape, shadows and textures.

- Now shift focus to your inner experiences. Can you name a feeling or emotion? What thoughts can you notice? Is there anything in your body that you have an urge to act on, such as hunger, thirst, an itch or stiffness?

- Finally shift your attention to a wider perspective. Can you hold awareness of multiple aspects of experience at once? Can you allow physical sensations, sounds, thoughts, emotions and visual stimuli to be present at the same time?

- Keep your attention wide as you reflect on these experiences. Use this big picture information to help you make a choice about where is most helpful to direct your attention next.

When Callum notices that he's getting stuck in an over-focused mind, he could try shifting his attention to focus on different aspects of his experience. He could also try setting a timer to remind him to take regular rests and breaks. Simple strategies like filling a water bottle and having it to hand might help keep him hydrated and also provide an opportunity to pause and notice the sensations of cool water in his mouth and the satisfaction of quenching his thirst.

In meetings, Callum can expand his attention to keep in mind his value of the relationship with his partners, alongside getting the task completed and agreed. He could try pausing to notice the sound of colleagues' voices, their body language and reactions, and allow more time to listen and ask questions. We talk more about how to build relationships in *Chapter 10*.

3.5 Practising mindfulness

Being open and observing involves developing skills in mindfulness, where we learn to pay attention to the present moment, without judging or trying to change our experience. To develop mindfulness skills, many people benefit from regular daily practice. However, this doesn't have to take a lot of time. Just a few minutes each day can help you to feel more aware and better able to cope with difficult thoughts and feelings.

Mindfulness: facts and myths

Here's our quick guide to what mindfulness is, and what it isn't:

Mindfulness is...	Mindfulness is not...
✔ Noticing and describing thoughts, feelings, body sensations, and what's around you with interest and curiosity	✘ Making your mind go blank, or trying to get rid of difficult thoughts or experiences
✔ Improving your ability to focus and to develop flexible attention to different parts of your experience	✘ Only beneficial after many hours of silent practice
✔ Learning to observe and respond to thoughts and difficult feelings with acceptance and kindness	✘ Intense focus on your breath whilst blocking out distressing parts of experience
✔ Stepping back rather than feeling overwhelmed by your experiences and being able to choose how to respond	✘ Learning to never have negative thoughts again
✔ Allowing your mind to recognise and appreciate moments of contentment and joy	✘ Something that you can judge yourself as 'good' or 'bad' at

3.6 Practising your Open and Observe skills

There are many mindfulness practices which can help you to develop your **Open and Observe** skills. There are helpful audio tracks available online (for example, those at https://insighttimer.com/drleedavid) that you can use to guide these practices.

If you don't feel able to commit to even a short daily mindfulness practice, there are also many ways to bring **Open and Observe** skills into our daily lives, which can help you to shift out of automatic pilot and become more present.

Paying attention to daily activities

Doing any everyday activity with a little more focus and awareness can be an opportunity to practise mindfulness. This might also help you appreciate these routine tasks and experience a sense of flow or contentment as you carry them out. Why not try one of the following examples?

- Notice the warmth and refreshing flow of water as you take a shower and breathe in the smell of your favourite shampoo or shower gel.

- When brushing your teeth, become aware of the sounds and the physical sensations on your teeth, gums and tongue as you move the toothbrush around your mouth.

- Notice your body moving as you carry out any form of activity or exercise, becoming aware of your feet on the ground, your legs moving, and the stretch through different muscles as you shift posture.

- Focus on the person that you are talking to, giving them the benefit of your full attention.

- When you get home from work, take a moment to connect with your partner, family or people around you, by pausing and paying attention as you smile and greet them warmly, or touch their arm.

- Pause to make eye contact, smile, and say thank you to the shop worker, or to the delivery driver who's bringing you a parcel or a takeaway meal.

Try the following Mindful Daily Activities:

EXERCISE: Mindful eating and drinking

Prepare by getting yourself something to eat or drink – it can be anything, from a glass of water to a raisin or a piece of chocolate.

Reach out slowly and pick up the food or drink. Notice how it feels in your hand: the weight, temperature and texture against your skin.

Slowly lift it towards your mouth. Pause to notice any smell before tasting it. Then take a small sip or place the food on your tongue. Hold it in your mouth for a short while, noticing the sensations, taste and temperature in your mouth.

Pause for a few seconds before you swallow and then feel the sensations as the food or drink moves down your throat.

Take another sip or bite and see if you can notice something different about the experience this time. Imagine that you had never tasted it before. How might you describe it to someone else?

Can you bring a little more mindful awareness to your experience when you eat or drink during the day?

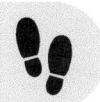

EXERCISE: Mindful walking

Take a short walk, outside or inside, using your five senses to be more aware of physically moving your body.

Take time to look at your surroundings. Can you notice something you haven't seen before? What colours or shapes are there?

What sounds can you notice? Can you hear the sound of your footsteps as you walk, the rustling of your clothes, the breeze in your ears, or your own breath?

Can you taste or smell anything?

What can you feel or touch? Notice the sensation of your feet in contact with the ground. Try making each step slow and deliberate, gradually shifting weight as you move, and paying attention to the many tiny sensations in your feet and legs.

When you find yourself getting distracted, congratulate yourself for becoming aware of this, and simply shift your attention back to the physical sensations of walking.

EXERCISE: Mindful listening

Take a moment to focus on one or more sounds. You could play a favourite piece of music or open the window and listen to the sounds outside.

Close your eyes and notice what sounds you can become aware of. What's the loudest sound you can hear? How about the quietest?

If you are listening to music, pay attention to the different instruments and any vocals and notice how these change throughout the piece. If you have heard the song before, can you notice anything new about it? Try noticing how often a particular sound or lyric repeats itself through the track.

Remain as focused as you can for one song. If you find your mind wandering, just gently and kindly bring your attention back to the music.

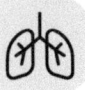

EXERCISE: Mindful breathing

Sit comfortably with your eyes closed or take a soft focus in front of you. Breathe in and then allow a long sigh as you exhale slowly. Let your body settle and start to feel heavier.

Start to notice your breathing. You might be aware of air moving through your nostrils or across your upper lip, or at the back of your throat. Maybe you feel the rise and fall of your chest or the gentle movement of your belly up and down with each breath.

Allow your awareness to rest gently on that place. There's no need to change or force the breath. Just a light touch, keeping your awareness on where you feel the rhythmic movement of breath in your body.

Perhaps wish yourself well as you take a few moments to practise self-care during your day. And when you find your mind wandering, as it will inevitably do at times, just gently bring it back to the breath with kindness and patience, recognising that each time we do this, is a moment of awareness.

Kayla, Practice Manager: *"I have so many different jobs to get through each day, and I find it hard to focus on one at a time. My mind keeps wandering onto the next task, or I'm interrupted by one of the team with an urgent problem, and it's hard to get back on track. Even when someone is talking to me, I find that my mind drifts away from the conversation. I'm thinking about all the other things I have to do or worrying about something that happened the day before. I keep having to ask the person to repeat what they are saying, and I'm sure my team are starting to notice. It's getting difficult to get anything done!*

Kayla decides to try a few minutes of daily mindfulness to see if this helps her focus on tasks at work. She chooses to practise using her five senses to pay attention to her daily shower for 3 minutes each morning. She notices the sensations of the water, the smell of her favourite shampoo, and the sounds of the water spray.

At lunchtime, she decides to try a 10 minute mindful walk to get some fresh air and focus her mind after a busy morning. She focuses on the feeling of each foot moving on the ground in turn. She looks around and notices the sky and the colour of the leaves in a tree, and the sounds of the traffic and the wind gently rustling in her ears.

After a few weeks of practice, Kayla finds it easier to keep her attention focused during work as well. If she finds her attention wandering in meetings, she takes a slow breath and then comes back to the present moment, noticing the sound of people's voices, the physical sensations of holding a pen in her fingers, or looking carefully at people's faces and expressions. She finds that brief mindfulness makes work feel more fulfilling and manageable and encourages her to appreciate and enjoy taking breaks and rests when needed.

3.7 Understanding our reactions

An important skill in using brief mindfulness to cope with difficult experiences is to give a name or a label to each different part of our experience. This process of 'Noticing and Naming' helps us to step back and feel less caught up by particular patterns of thoughts or emotions.

The 'low road' and the 'high road' of the stress response

When faced by a stressful life experience we can process this through two different pathways. Our initial response to stress is often via the 'low road'. This involves activation of parts of the brain such as the amygdala, which detects a threat to our survival and triggers the sympathetic 'fight, flight or freeze' reaction. This pathway allows us to respond quickly to potential danger but also leads to feelings of anxiety and frustration, and if overused, can lead to chronic stress and burnout.

An alternative is to process the experience using the 'high road'. This involves different areas of the brain, such as the prefrontal cortex, which can process information before relaying it to the amygdala. This pathway is slower, allowing time for a more thorough analysis of the situation, and enables us to take a more realistic and thoughtful response to varying levels of threat.

If we get stuck in a 'low road' response, our habitual reaction to challenging life experiences is to activate the amygala and trigger the fight, flight or freeze response, leading to anxiety, tension and irritability.

An alternative is to use **Open and Observe** skills to strengthen the 'high road' pathways so that these become our new default reaction. We can do this simply by improving our awareness and our ability to notice and name our inner experiences. It's not necessary to get stuck in a mental debate about which is the 'right' way to view a particular problem. The process of acknowledging and labelling our experiences may be enough to engage the prefontal cortex, widen our perspective and reduce the stress response.

EXERCISE: Notice the NOW

Next time you are starting to feel stressed or tense, practise noticing and labelling your inner experiences, by noticing the NOW:

- **N**otice and name your thoughts and feelings: *I'm worrying about the next patient on my list. I feel a tightness in my stomach. I notice I am anxious and tense.*

- **O**bserve your outer body and the world around, using your five senses: *I can feel my feet on the floor and my fingers typing resting on the computer keyboard. I can see a bird flying outside the window. I can hear the noise of people talking in the next room.*

- **W**hat matters? Decide what's most important for you to focus on and move to do this with your full attention: *It's important that I concentrate on the phone call that I'm about to make. I can listen and pay attention so I am responsive and can use my knowledge and experience.*

Using a CBT framework

A CBT framework offers a structure for making sense of our experiences by breaking them down into five areas (see figure below):

- *Thoughts, beliefs and thinking patterns*: these include the words, stories, ideas and images that arise inside our mind and help us understand the world.

- *Feelings and emotions* such as anger, fear, joy and guilt.

- *In the body*: physical sensations may arise for many different reasons, including sensations from what we are touching physically and symptoms due to illness or injury, or basic needs such as hunger, thirst and fatigue. Physical reactions often also arise when we experience an emotion, such as tightness in the chest or neck or a racing heart with feelings of anxiety.

- *Behaviour, actions and urges*: this involves what you choose to do – what actions you take. Of the five areas, behaviour is the one that we have most control over. It is far easier to control our behaviour than our thoughts or feelings. For example, you might be able to notice the urge to carry out a behaviour before you actually do it – and then decide if it's helpful or not.

- *Situation, environment and triggers* in the external world. External factors such as where you are, who you are with, what your life experience has been so far, and what you are paying attention to, will influence how you feel and react at any given moment.

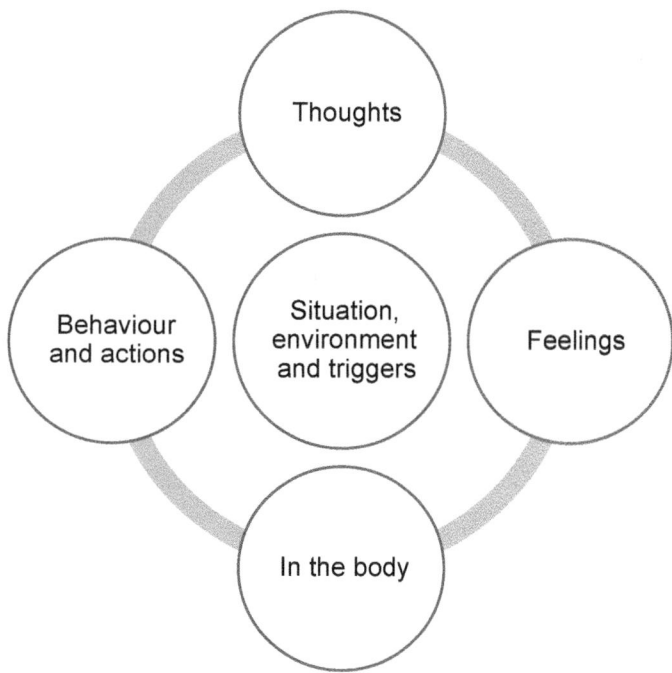

Links between areas of the CBT framework

Links between areas of the CBT framework can create both negative and positive cycles. If we are feeling hopeful or energised, we may respond to a difficult patient with patience, kindness and understanding, and avoid confrontation whilst continuing to be assertive and fair as we support ourselves and our colleagues. On another day, when feeling low, irritable or frustrated, we may respond very differently, leading to a distressing experience of conflict, which results in a complaint that takes many months to resolve. The table below shows some examples of different types of emotions and how these can influence our thoughts and behaviour.

FEELINGS	THOUGHTS	BODY SENSATIONS	URGES
Joyful Happy Excited Determined Hopeful	I am respected I am valued I can cope I am motivated This is interesting	Smiling Energetic Strong Lightness Vitality	To move To do exercise To engage socially To keep trying To have fun
Peaceful Calm Relaxed Content	I am cared about I am fulfilled I am safe This is enjoyable	Relaxed muscles Warmth Unhurried Soft	To rest To hug someone To read To listen to music
Angry Irritable Frustrated Hostile Fed up	This is wrong They are disrespectful This is unacceptable It's not fair I feel rejected	Headache Neck pain Clenched fists Hot (head, face, neck) Tingling/prickles	To argue To lash out To shout To break something To move violently
Anxious Fearful Worried Nervous Panicky	This is risky Something may go wrong I might make a mistake I can't cope I'm not safe	Tense, fidgety, shaky Tight chest Butterflies, nausea Racing heart Sweaty palms	To ask for reassurance To pace around To escape To over-plan To check something
Embarrassed Ashamed Jealous Lonely	I look foolish They are unkind I'm being excluded I'm not important	Burning Numbness Chest discomfort Flushed cheeks	To retaliate To eat something unhealthy To withdraw To self-sabotage
Sad Low Guilty Despondent Despairing	I am useless I'm a terrible practitioner I can't be bothered Nothing will improve What's the point?	Fatigue, lethargy Aches and pains Heaviness Slowness Poor sleep	To give up To avoid eye contact To stop socializing To lie down and rest To stop working
Other feelings:	Other thoughts:	Other body sensations:	Other urges

EXERCISE: Using the CBT framework to reflect on your experiences

Think about a time that you recently experienced a difficult feeling or emotion. Don't pick anything overwhelming – perhaps a time that you felt slightly stressed, nervous, irritable or fed up.

Use the five areas of the CBT framework to map out your experiences:

Situation, environment and triggers: What was happening? Where were you? Who was involved? What were the triggers for any difficult emotions? What other background experiences were relevant?	
Thoughts, beliefs and thinking patterns: What thoughts went through your mind? Why was this important? What was the worst that might happen? Did you notice any images?	
Feelings: What feelings or emotions can you notice, either at the time, or afterwards as you reflect?	
In the body: What was happening in your body? What physical sensations can you become aware of?	
Behaviour and actions: What did you do (or have the urge to do)? What was the long-term and short-term impact of this action? Did you avoid doing anything?	
Observe and reflect: What can you notice or learn about this experience? What one action could you choose that might help you cope more effectively?	

Inger, Salaried GP: *"I usually like my patients and enjoy my job, but lately I've found myself getting increasingly drained from all their demands. By the end of the day, I'm exhausted and I'm starting to lose my empathy. Many of my patients have emotional and mental health problems, and I've always enjoyed this part of the role, but more recently I'm increasingly tired and I've started to dread it when people tell me they are feeling low or anxious. I'm getting really overwhelmed, especially during a long and busy day."*

Inger could use a CBT framework to label and understand her experiences, helping her to shift from the 'low road' stress response, by engaging the 'high road' pathways of her brain, where she is more aware and able to step back and to recognise and process what's happening.

Situation, environment and triggers: What was happening? Where were you? Who was involved? What were the triggers for any difficult emotions? What other background experiences were relevant?	Yesterday afternoon, a patient had a long list of problems. Usually, I'm fairly patient but this time it felt like more than I could cope with. It was a busy day and I had been duty doctor all morning. I had lunch at my desk and then the first patient of the afternoon brought out a ridiculous long list of ailments. It was too much!
Thoughts, beliefs and thinking patterns: What thoughts went through your mind? Why was this important? What was the worst that might happen? Did you notice any images?	I had a lot of thoughts such as: I can't cope with this! I'm going to be running late for the rest of the day. I'll never make this person happy. I can't cope with this job. No one is ever satisfied. What's the point?
Feelings: What feelings or emotions can you notice, either at the time, or afterwards as you reflect?	I felt frustrated and stressed, and very irritable.

In the body:
What was happening in your body? What physical sensations can you become aware of?

My face felt hot, and my chest felt tight. I started getting a headache.

Behaviour and actions:
What did you do (or have the urge to do)? What was the long-term and short-term impact of this action? Did you avoid doing anything?

I wanted to yell at her to just come with one problem and not to waste my time! I felt like jumping up and running out of the room. I was very short with the patient and rushed through her problems, even though one of them was quite serious. Afterwards, I started worrying that I might have missed something or that she might complain about me.

Observe and reflect:
What can you notice or learn about this experience? What one action could you choose that might help you cope more effectively?

I can see that I was exhausted, and it would have been better to take more time at lunch to take a break. I don't want to miss something important, and I want to retain my interest and empathy. I could also learn some ways to cope with people who bring a list of problems – one of my colleagues is good at being assertive – perhaps I could ask her for advice.

3.8 Stepping back and making space

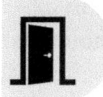

No matter how distressing they are, it's impossible to simply 'get rid of' difficult thoughts and feelings. An alternative, which may seem counter-intuitive at first, is to be *willing* to experience whatever comes up, allowing the experience to be there and making some inner space for difficulties and discomfort. This is a little like becoming Dr Who's Tardis – we become bigger on the inside!

We can stop struggling to get rid of problems we cannot solve and focus on living the life we choose, in spite of or alongside negative thoughts and feelings. You can use **Open and Observe** skills to help with this. You could try stepping back and simply noticing that the uncomfortable thought or feeling is present, and then give it a bit of room to pass in its own time, without fighting to feel differently, shut it out or avoid it, which often only makes things worse.

Remember, what you can control is your behaviour – what you choose to do; and your attention – where you choose to focus your awareness. So, you can make choices to behave in ways that are meaningful and consistent with your values, no matter what arises internally, and you can take difficult thoughts and feelings along with you on the journey.

Coping with strong emotions

We can use **Open and Observe** as useful tools to cope with high levels of emotion. When we are hit by an emotional storm, such as fear, anger or shame, we need to find ways to keep ourselves safe and grounded, whilst waiting for better weather. The process of making space within can help us to find ways to allow difficult feelings to arise inside, but without letting these pull us into making choices or decisions that move us away from our inner **Guide** and what matters most.

Steady yourself with your five senses

Next time you are hit by a strong wave of emotion, use your five senses to create a feeling of stability, steady yourself, and make space inside, whilst you engage your 'high road' pathways. It's not necessary to use all five – just pick whatever seems most helpful and relevant at the time.

- What can you see around you? Notice at least one colour – can you find two or three objects with the same colour? Repeat with another colour.

- What sounds can you hear around you? What are the loudest and quietest sounds?

- What are you touching with your hands or skin? Exaggerate the sensations by gently moving your body. Push your feet into the ground, wriggle in your seat on the chair, push your back against the cushion behind you, reach your arms upwards and stretch through your shoulders and back.

- What can you smell or taste? Pause and take a small sip of your drink or a mouthful of food. Hold it in your mouth and become aware of the flavour and sensation on your tongue.

- Are there any sensations inside your body? Can you label these descriptively, such as noticing warmth, aching, softness, tightness, fluttering or tension?

- What's going through your mind? What thoughts can you notice? How busy is your mind? What type of thoughts are you having – are they realistic and balanced, or fearful and catastrophic?

- What emotions can you notice? Where can you find these in your body?

- Finish by allowing yourself to breathe out slowly with a long gentle sigh. Now, connect with what's most important for you to be doing at this moment. Move back to doing this with your full attention. Can you keep focused on this activity, whilst allowing any inner experiences to also remain present?

Playing an inner game of chess

We can think of our inner world like a game of chess, with our thoughts and feelings represented by the pieces on the board. We often get into a battle between different perspectives. "Oh no, did I make a mistake today…? No, I'm sure it was fine… I need to get rid of these feelings of anxiety… I will just check once more or ask my colleague for reassurance…"

The problem with an inner game of chess is that you are playing yourself, so whichever side wins, you will also lose.

Instead of battling harder to try to convince yourself or to 'win', we can instead engage with the 'high road' and simply **observe** the game. We can see ourselves as the board itself, allowing the complex game of thoughts and feelings to play out, but without wanting either side to win or lose. Or you can take the perspective of an interested spectator, who is captivated by watching the twists and turns of the game, no matter who wins.

From this wider perspective we have more capacity to see the big picture, and this can help in decision-making and managing complex situations. Stepping back and taking time to reflect on all the information might just help us pick up a rare diagnosis, or create space to take a breath, practise some self-care and make a cup of tea before getting back to work.

Following your Guide when life is uncomfortable

Being able to cope with all the difficult thoughts, feelings, urges and all the discomfort that comes with being human, brings many benefits and a sense of freedom. And it helps if you continue following your inner **Guide**, doing the things you know are important, and becoming the person you want to be, despite any difficulties that pop up on the way.

You could think of this as surfing a wave and staying on your board, feeling the thrill of riding over it. Or going over a bump in the road and continuing to stay on track and doing what matters, even if you experience problems or negative thoughts and feelings.

 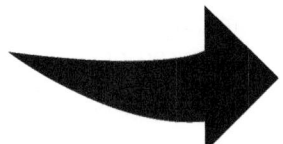

What is most important to me?

EXERCISE: Following your Guide through discomfort

Think of a time when you felt apprehensive about doing something but did it anyway because it was important. This could be a time you spoke up for someone, completed a sports challenge, sat an exam, or went into a new situation.

Describe the situation: What happened? What did you do?	
What uncomfortable thoughts and feelings did you overcome in order to do this?	
What important values were being met? Were you following your **Guide**?	
How does it feel, right now in this moment, when you think about this?	
What was the long-term impact of overcoming difficult thoughts and feelings?	

3.9 Finding enjoyment and contentment

We can also use **Open and Observe** to become more aware of any moments of contentment, joy and happiness that naturally arise through our day. Because of the 'negativity bias' of the brain, there is a tendency to focus on negative experiences and ignore what's gone well.

Instead, we can take time to actively focus our attention on things that we can appreciate or feel grateful for. This isn't about ignoring or shutting out problems, but about making space to recognise and acknowledge positive experiences alongside difficulties. This can help to build a sense of resilience and hopefulness and strengthen relationships with people around us.

Which environments and activities make it easier for you to appreciate where you are and what is going on around you?

- Do you get a sense of freedom or peacefulness outdoors? In a woodland? By the sea? Looking down from a mountain or a hilltop? Picture this in your mind.

- Do you notice smells when you are in a freshly cut field? Holding a bunch of flowers? In a coffee shop? When cooking your favourite dish?

- Do you notice sounds and different instruments when you are listening to music? When you wake up early and hear birdsong? When the wind passes through the trees?

- Do you appreciate touch when you sink into the sofa? When a family member gives you a hug? When you wear something soft? When you stroke a pet?

- When do you appreciate taste? When having your first drink of the day? When eating something rich and spicy?

EXERCISE: Gratitude and appreciation

Bring to mind a sight that you appreciate visually. Perhaps it's the sight of someone's face, a beautiful view, or a building that you love to look at. Notice the colours, shadows, shapes and movement. Breathe in and allow yourself to rest in gentle gratitude for being able to use your vision to experience the amazing world of colour and shape.

Now allow something to come to mind that has a taste that you enjoy. Allow yourself to gently savour the flavour, smell and texture of this food or drink. Take a moment to think of all the people who have been involved in growing the ingredients, harvesting, transporting, packaging and selling. And send appreciation for their efforts and wish everyone well who has been involved in this chain that leads to you.

And now the sense of touch. Bring to mind a physical experience that you appreciate. Perhaps it's the feeling of water streaming onto you in a shower, a pet that you love to stroke, or a soft material that feels warm and calming. You might offer yourself a gentle touch by stroking your own arm from the shoulder down to the hand. Or place a hand over your heart, noticing the warmth and the pressure, and sending yourself kindness and well-wishing. Acknowledge and offer yourself thanks and appreciation for all the efforts that you make each day.

And now just gently bring your awareness back to your body, sitting, your seat on the chair, your feet on the ground. Take a breath in and allow a gentle slow sigh as you finish the practice.

Aftab, GP Registrar: *"I had to gather patient and colleague feedback. Nearly all of it was positive, commenting on all the things I had done well and saying that I am thorough, thoughtful and a good doctor. But there was one negative comment from a patient that said I was running late, I hadn't listened well, and they would not want to see me again. Despite all the praise and positive feedback, all I could think about afterwards was this one negative comment. I found it hard to sleep for worrying that I had upset someone. I wish I could feel happier because most of the comments were very supportive."*

Aftab could use a regular gratitude practice to help him pay attention to the positive experiences in his life, which will help to create a sense of balance, and not get overly hooked into negative experiences.

Aftab decides to take 5 minutes at the end of each day to focus on something that he appreciated during the day. He decides to keep a note of these in a journal to help him remember them more easily:

- An elderly patient smiled and said thanks very much for my help today. I felt really proud that I was able to help her deal with a complicated problem.

- I had a nice lunch and chatted with my Trainer today. It was nice to connect with her and relax a little.

- My wife sent me a video of my youngest son taking his first step! It was lovely to see this, and I felt really proud.

Chapter summary: Open and Observe

- Using **Open and Observe** skills involves stepping out of automatic pilot and becoming more aware of your own reactions, without getting caught in habitual patterns of unhelpful behaviour.

- **Notice the NOW** helps us focus on the present moment and observe our reactions, before choosing the most helpful activity to move onto next.

- Increased awareness and labelling of our inner reactions can help to develop the 'high road' pathway for understanding and processing stressful life experiences.

- A CBT framework can help to make sense of our experiences by breaking them down into thoughts, feelings, body sensations, actions and the environment.

- We can use our five senses to help us pause and find a sense of stability when hit by strong or difficult emotions.

- We can also use **Open and Observe** to become more aware of the moments of contentment, joy and happiness that naturally arise through each day.

Final thoughts

What are the most important messages for you from this chapter?

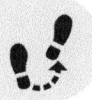

Take an action step

What are your next steps? What actions will you take as a result of reading this chapter?

What practical steps can you take to help you **Observe** and be more **Open** to the present moment?

04 Wise Mind

- Do you make reasoned, thoughtful decisions in your work and personal life, or do you battle with inner doubt, uncertainty or mental recriminations?

- Do you get stuck in negative mental loops, churning over problems, mistakes and regrets, or worrying about disastrous possible future outcomes?

- Are you able to keep a balanced, flexible perspective, or do you get hooked into habitual negative ways of looking at the world and reacting to situations?

- Do you want to listen more to your **Wise Mind** and take wise action? Keep reading…

4.1 What is Wise Mind?

Our mind comprises the many thoughts, beliefs, stories and images which allow us to make sense of the world. It is also influenced by our background, training, education, attitudes and personality, and by events in our lives and the people around us, both past and present. The mind represents our inner world and is invisible to others, although the *effects* are visible, as it will influence how we feel, behave and react.

Wise Mind involves balancing logic and emotions: using our reasoning and evaluating skills, coupled with our capacity to feel emotions and empathise with the feelings of others. Listening to **Wise Mind** involves looking at the big picture and thinking flexibly, adapting our perspective to meet new challenges, and looking for ways to resolve difficulties.

In this chapter we look at how developing and listening to your **Wise Mind** can build on the previous steps we have discussed, to help manage stress, build resilience, and protect against burnout or mental ill-health. In this chapter we will look at some ways to:

- Notice any **thought patterns** that are unhelpful, create distress, or which get in the way of leading a full and meaningful life.

- Notice the point at which you have a **choice** about which thoughts to listen to, how to react and what action to take.

- **Recognise and 'unhook'** from negative thoughts without struggling to get rid of them, using techniques such as noticing, labelling, shifting attention, and choosing how you respond.

- Learn some skills to **respond wisely to urges** linked to strong emotions and how to choose actions that are helpful in challenging situations.

Matthew, GP Registrar: Matthew has been experiencing stress and low mood for some months. He has been working on structuring positive activities during his week and has found this helpful. With the support of his Trainer, he has also made progress with building his confidence at work. However, he still has a major problem with completing e-portfolio entries.

"I find it hard to focus and I get very self-critical about the entries that I write. I often procrastinate and put off getting started, and then I get stressed because I have so much to catch up on. When I sit down to try and write any reflective entries, I find it hard to concentrate because I have so many intrusive thoughts about how useless I am, and how my educational supervisor will read it and realise that I'm really incompetent. My mind gets so caught up with all these thoughts that I can't decide what to write, so I end up doing a very short entry that I know is not really a high standard, or just walking away and leaving it even longer before I get started."

Neelam, Practice Nurse: Neelam has always enjoyed her job, but lately has been experiencing increasing anxiety after seeing patients.

"I get really anxious after a clinic thinking whether I might have done something wrong, made a mistake, or somehow offended one of the patients. I get horrible feelings of shame as I remember what I did or said and wonder if I could have done it differently or better. I get so stuck in my mind, it's hard to get on with my day afterwards, and I keep forgetting to do things that are important. I'm getting quite snappy and irritable with colleagues and with my husband when I get home because I'm so preoccupied. I've started having a few glasses of wine every night because otherwise I can't get to sleep with all these thoughts whirling round in my head."

PAUSE AND REFLECT: Patterns of thinking

What is your reaction to the two examples? Are there any thought patterns that seem familiar to you? What is the impact of the thought patterns on Matthew and Neelam in terms of their emotional reactions and behaviour? What might be the long-term consequences?

4.2 We are not our thoughts

Thoughts are mental events that pop up in the mind. Like clouds passing across the sky, thoughts will come and go, and can change in different situations. It's possible for the same person to have both positive and negative thoughts about the same issue on different days. You can even deliberately choose to think something that's not true, such as "I have green hair" (or whatever colour hair you don't have!).

Despite the transient nature of thoughts, we often treat them as concrete facts. However, we can try to recognise that they are simply opinions, interpretations or assumptions, which may need to be updated when we learn new information. Remember, your mind is not always your friend. The thoughts that pop up can be exaggerated, unhelpful, critical and hurtful, and may lead you into spirals of negativity and low mood. But you are not your thoughts, and you don't have to believe or act on every single thought that you experience.

Whether accurate or exaggerated, your thoughts and beliefs can shape our reality by influencing the actions that you take. Whilst you cannot control the thoughts that pop into your mind, you can choose and control how you behave in response to your thoughts.

EXERCISE: Noticing thoughts	
Think of a difficult challenge that you have been facing recently. What types of negative thoughts tend to pop up in your mind?	
What feelings or emotions are linked to these thoughts?	
How do the thoughts affect your behaviour or actions? What do you have the urge to do when you are thinking this way?	
What might be the long-term effect of acting in this way?	
Notice your choices: What other choices do you have for your actions?	

4.3 Thoughts and emotions

Our thoughts are influenced by our emotions and mood. When we are feeling happy and upbeat, we are more likely to experience optimistic and positive thoughts, as if wearing rose-tinted glasses. Similarly, when we are feeling low, irritable or anxious, the lens can darken, and we may see the world in a more negative or gloomy light.

Experiencing powerful emotions can make us more likely to think in extreme or unhelpful ways and we may find it harder to find a balanced or rational perspective. Strong emotions make these negative thoughts *feel* convincing, even when they may be exaggerated, unrealistic or irrational. So, when we are in a state of rage, we might get stuck in thoughts that blame others, and when we are feeling anxious or panicky, we may be convinced by our terrifying thoughts predicting future catastrophes.

This is where **Wise Mind** comes in. Rather than following the same old patterns or choosing actions based on unhelpful thoughts, emotions or impulses, **Wise Mind** helps you get perspective, step back and walk the fine line that considers both logic and reasoning *and* your own feelings about the situation. This helps you make choices and take actions that work for you – and others – whatever context you are in.

4.4 Negative thinking patterns

At times, we have all experienced self-critical or defeatist thoughts. If we believe and buy into these thoughts, which are often long-standing and habitual, they can undermine our belief in ourselves and distort our view of the world. **Rumination** is when our minds get stuck repeatedly churning over and analysing past events, triggering emotions of guilt, regret and shame. We may also get trapped in a loop of **worry**, where our thoughts go forwards, constantly focusing on potential future problems and catastrophic outcomes.

Instead of going into automatic pilot and following these habitual thinking patterns, we can use **Open and Observe** to recognise when they are popping up and then choose a more balanced, helpful or Wise perspective, taking us in the direction of our inner **Guide**.

Difficult patients at your surgery

We can imagine our minds as being like a busy GP surgery. Our thoughts represent the many patients who show up to be seen each day and then leave again. Negative thoughts are like difficult patients who arrive at the surgery, complain about how long they have to wait to be seen, make unreasonable demands, and criticise the hard-working staff. They can be loud and dominating, and often bring negative emotions such as fear, anger, self-doubt and low mood.

How do we respond to these difficult thoughts when they show up at the surgery? On a bad day, we might react in less helpful ways, perhaps by getting angry, aggressive or confrontational. We may also try to avoid them, hiding in our room until they leave, because we fear confrontation, or we don't want to face their complaints and criticism.

An alternative approach is to acknowledge that the difficult patients have arrived, along with many uncomfortable emotions. We can't stop them from showing up, but we can choose how we respond when they arrive. We do not have to agree with their perspective or give in to their unreasonable demands. However, getting aggressive or trying to hide from them is equally unhelpful. Instead, we can calmly and assertively approach the situation, making choices about what is fair and realistic, whilst keeping our compassion for any distressing emotions that arise.

Thinking traps

Thinking traps involve common patterns of thoughts that can pull us into seeing the world in a negative way. The following table shows some common examples of thinking traps:

Thinking trap	Typical thoughts	Possible impact
Rumination and negative bias	*I shouldn't have...* *I really regret...* *I cringe when I picture myself...*	Low mood, demoralisation, shame, loss of confidence, withdrawal
Worry and catastrophic predictions	*What if....?* *The worst might happen...!* *What if my mistake causes permanent harm?*	Anxiety, stress, difficulty relaxing, over-preparing, checking, avoidance
Doubt and intolerance of uncertainty	*I must do the right thing* *I have to know the answer* *I need to be sure*	Worry, checking, reassurance-seeking, compulsive or obsessive behaviour, indecision
Perfectionism	*It must be absolutely right* *I should do this perfectly* *Mistakes are unacceptable*	Demanding behaviour, over-working, lack of delegation, repeating, procrastination
Self-criticism	*I am useless... incompetent... a failure.... selfish.... lazy...* *I'm not as good as others*	Loss of confidence, low mood, fatigue, avoiding challenges
Blaming or being critical of others	*They are incompetent!* *It's their fault* *She is completely unreasonable!*	Anger, irritability, lack of trust and teamwork, not listening to others' viewpoints

Permissive or emotional reasoning	*I know it's unhealthy, but it helps me relax…* *I can't stand feeling like this. I need a release…* *I just need to feel calm…*	Impulsive or addictive behaviour, over-eating, alcohol, self-sabotage

Observing our thinking patterns

The first step in using **Wise Mind** is to **notice** and **label** your thoughts, beliefs and thinking patterns, without judging them. This engages our 'high road' pathways (see *Section 3.7*) that we looked at in *Chapter 3*. We start to recognise and treat negative thoughts as opinions rather than facts. And it helps us to avoid getting entangled with any thinking traps before we slip into unhelpful patterns of behaviour and reactions. We might use one of the following labels:

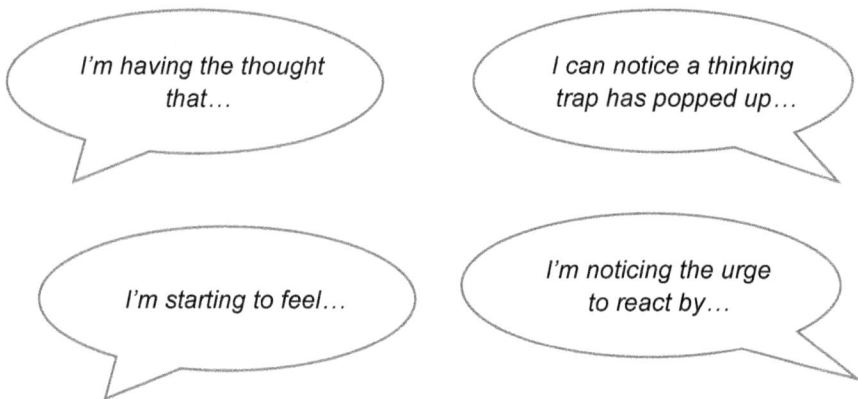

I'm having the thought that…

I can notice a thinking trap has popped up…

I'm starting to feel…

I'm noticing the urge to react by…

Noticing and labelling thoughts builds on other ways to be **Open and Observe** mindfully, which we introduced in *Chapter 3*. Using these strategies can help us to ride the wave of the urge to do something that takes us away from our values and instead choose actions that take us towards the rich, fulfilling life we seek.

PAUSE AND REFLECT: Noticing thinking traps

Do any of the thinking traps seem familiar? Complete the following table to start to recognise some of your own thinking patterns, urges and behaviours, in stressful or challenging situations. If you could press replay on the situation, at what point could you have done something different – made a different choice?

Thinking trap	Do you recognise this thinking trap? What situations does it arise in?	What thoughts come up? What emotions or behaviours are linked?	What's the impact or long-term effect of this thinking trap?	What different choices could you make?
Rumination and negative bias				
Worry and catastrophic predictions				
Doubt and intolerance of uncertainty				
Perfectionism				
Self-criticism				
Blaming or being critical of others				
Permissive or emotional reasoning				

Matthew says: "*I recognise many of these thinking traps – they pop up as soon as I sit down and start trying to do entries in my portfolio. I get a lot of self-critical thoughts about how useless I am and how the entries are not up to scratch. I can be quite perfectionist – I want it to be really good and it's hard to live up to such a high standard. I also get stuck in a lot of worry about the future – I start thinking that I'm going to fail, and I will never make it through my training to be a GP. Then I start worrying about how we will pay the mortgage if I'm not able to practise any more. All of these thoughts go round and round, and I can see that they are a big distraction from focusing on doing my written entries.*

The long-term impact of thinking like this is that it is getting in the way of my career! It's stopping me from doing my reflective entries to the best of my abilities and from making progress towards qualifying as a GP. I don't want to be thinking like this for every appraisal throughout the rest of my working life. I think the moment that I have a choice is when I sit down at the computer. I can get stuck in the usual negative thoughts in my mind, or I can make an effort to focus and pay attention to what I really want to do – which is to just get on with the entry as best I can."

Neelam says: *"I can recognise almost all of these thinking traps! I get stuck in worry about having done or said something wrong during the day, and I catastrophise about how serious the consequences might be, such as getting a complaint and losing my job. I also do a lot of rumination – going over and over my day, trying to pick out if I really did make a mistake or if everything is OK. Eventually I get tired and irritable, and I start to blame others. I find myself blaming the patient for being unreasonable, or I might get irritable and argue with colleagues, or with my husband for not saying exactly the right thing when I tell him how I'm feeling. I also can recognise quite a bit of permissive reasoning – I tell myself that after a busy day I 'need' a glass of wine, and end up drinking most of the bottle, or eating way more than I really want to, and it feels good at the time, but afterwards I feel bloated and guilty.*

One point that I can make a different choice is when I feel the urge to reach for another glass of wine. If I can pause and recognise that this a moment of choice, it might help me to step out of autopilot and bring on board my Wise Mind, and then decide what's really best for me in the longer term."

4.5 Let go of the struggle

Even though you might recognise that some of your thinking patterns are unhelpful, it can be hard to change them. As much as you might wish to rid yourself of your negative thoughts, it's simply not possible to just stop yourself from having thoughts that you don't want! Trying to push away negative thoughts takes a lot of effort, is tiring, can leave you feeling frustrated, and takes your attention away from doing other things that matter to you. And sometimes the harder you try to get rid of difficult thoughts and feelings, the stronger they can grow.

Instead, you could let the thought or emotion be there for a while – acknowledge it, allow it – even make some space for it, and accept it. This doesn't mean that you have to agree with the thought or do what it says, especially if this behaviour is unhelpful for you. Instead, letting go of the struggle to stop thinking negatively gives the thought or the emotion less power and intensity and may make it easier to make Wise choices, even if the thought or emotion is still present.

The key is to be aware of your thoughts and feelings and catch them at the point at which you can make a choice about what action to take in response to them. We can 'freeze frame' and create a tiny pause – just long enough for **Wise Mind** to step in and influence our actions and the outcome. This will help surf the urge to carry out unhelpful actions, which may be driven by strong negative emotions.

So how do you allow a thought to be present without struggling? There are many ways to do this. Why not try out some of the following techniques and see if you find any of them helpful?

Find an ARC to bridge difficult experiences

An arc is a beautiful shape, which symbolises a rainbow or a bridge taking you from where you are to where you want to go. You might find it helpful to conjure up your own ARC image to help you respond to unwanted intrusive thoughts:

- **Acknowledge the thought and feeling:** Pause and take a moment to 'freeze frame', and notice and name what thoughts and feelings have arisen: *"I'm feeling tense, agitated, stressed or anxious... I'm imagining the worst-case scenario... I'm worrying about..."*

- **Recognise the urge to react:** Take a breath in and a long, slow exhale from your belly, and turn your attention to any urges to take action. What is your instinctive, automatic reaction to these uncomfortable thoughts and feelings? *"I'm having the urge to escape from this stress... I'm feeling like yelling and throwing something right now!"*

- **Choose your Wise response:** Take another slow exhale and choose what will be your wisest response. What is most likely to be helpful? What Towards actions are in line with your values and the person you really want to be, even when you are experiencing discomfort and distress?

Find the big picture perspective

Wise Mind takes a big picture view of any situation which takes into account the context, our wider values, and many other factors that may not be obvious at first glance.

It can help to create some imagery for this. Can you imagine that you are standing high up in the mountains, flying high in a helicopter, soaring like a bird in the wind, or floating with the clouds in the sky, and looking down at the vast expansive view below? As you rise upwards to take this perspective, you continue to experience your thoughts and feelings, but they may seem less intense and overwhelming. This can help you to think more clearly and flexibly and adapt your reactions to match each new challenge that you face.

PAUSE AND REFLECT: Wise perspective

Think of a recent disagreement you had with a colleague or family member. Pick a scenario that does not trigger extreme or high levels of emotion, but where you might benefit from expanding your perspective.

Start by asking yourself: What frustrates or distresses me about this situation? What is my initial reaction or perspective from close up or at ground level?

Now choose your favourite imagery and imagine yourself rising above the situation to get a wider perspective. What would the view look like from up here? Now ask yourself the following questions:

Your perspective	What happens as you widen your perspective and see the view from above? Can you notice any new information?	
Other people's perspective	From your new perspective, is it possible to notice how things might appear to others who are involved? What might be their values, needs or motivations?	
A neutral observer	How might this seem to someone neutral and who is not emotionally involved with the situation?	
Shifting time perspectives	How might this seem 6 months from now? How about in a year? What about in 5 or 10 years? Does this change your perspective on the problem?	
Wise Mind	Pause and reflect: What would be the best thing (for you and others) in this situation? What's your Wisest perspective? What Wise Actions can you take?	

4.6 'Defuse' from unhelpful thoughts

It's easy to get caught up in our mind and start to see our thoughts as being absolute fact, especially when emotions are high. Cognitive defusion is a process of stepping back and learning to notice thoughts, allowing them to come and go, recognising that they are just one perspective or opinion. As we become more aware of the process of thinking, we are better able to reflect and problem-solve before taking any action.

We have already introduced some techniques to help 'defuse' from unhelpful thoughts, such as to notice and name your thoughts and feelings. Here are some of our other favourite strategies:

Scroll past social media

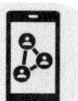

Try viewing your thoughts as a status update on social media. If you are scrolling through Facebook, Twitter or Instagram and you come to a post that's negative or unhelpful, you have a choice. You might decide to stop and read it, perhaps start disagreeing and arguing with whoever made the post. But this may give more time and attention to the negative post than you would really like and prevents you doing other things. It can also stir up negative emotions and reactions.

Another option is to simply continue scrolling. Ignore the negative post and move on to do something more interesting and important. Similarly, you can choose to scroll past negative thoughts. Next time a negative or unhelpful thought pops up into your mind, try scrolling past as if it were a social media post.

Say to yourself: "I'm having another Facebook update!" or "My Mind is Tweeting that…" or think of it like an annoying pop-up advert. Remember, you don't have to click on the advert, spend time engaging with the negative post or react to the thought.

Can you simply move on and do something else more important?

Bad weather thoughts

Try viewing negative thoughts and feelings like a temporary change in the weather. Clouds may come and it may rain for a while, but sooner or later, the clouds will pass, and the sun will come out again, so it's not necessary to take the thoughts too seriously.

The 'bad weather forecast' thoughts are saying that I'm going to mess this up!

Thoughts on a TV screen

Imagine that your thoughts and images are being played on a TV screen. If you get too hooked into your mind, it's like watching in full colour on the big screen in a cinema, with your thoughts being broadcast on surround sound.

Now, imagine the screen shrinks down to the size of your mobile phone. The movie and soundtrack are still playing, but it's much smaller and quieter and you are more aware of the rest of your environment. You can put the phone in your pocket and continue with your day, even if the movie is still playing.

Change the voice

Try saying a negative thought really slowly, or in a silly high-pitched voice. You could also try singing the thought, in your head or out loud, using a voice from a character in a movie or cartoon, or even try using a voice-changing app to play back the thought on your phone. Notice how using a different voice helps to separate you from the content of the thought, making it feel less believable. This is a process of defusion.

This technique is best used for annoying or niggly recurrent worries that keep popping up over and over again. It's less helpful for more distressing or traumatic thoughts or memories.

Write it out

Writing the thought on a sticky note, or on a computer screen, can also help to create a sense of defusion. You can play with the size, font and colour, and see if this changes how you relate to the thought.

I'm having the thought that...

Instead of saying to yourself, "This is a disaster, I'm going to fail this exam…", describe the thought: "I'm having a thought that 'This is a disaster and I'm worried I'm going to fail this exam…'". By doing this you are taking one step further away and seeing the thought as just a thought or an opinion, not an absolute irrefutable fact.

Next time Matthew sits down to complete an entry in his portfolio, he could try looking at the big picture and take a 'helicopter view' rather than getting caught up in the negative automatic thoughts that arise in his mind.

"I like the idea of imagining myself rising up above the computer and watching from up in the clouds. From up here, I can see how this will benefit my career in the long run, even if I don't feel comfortable doing it right now. It feels less stressful and it's a bit easier to get on with the entries. I'm less caught up in the negative predictions and worries.

I also like the image of seeing my thoughts as annoying pop-ups on the screen. When they appear, I don't have to click on them, because this just makes them multiply. I can move them to the side of the screen and just keep working."

TAKE ACTION: Defusing from unhelpful thoughts

Take another look at the strategies we have suggested for 'defusing' from negative or unhelpful thoughts and mindsets. Which of these seem most useful for you? How and when can you commit to trying to use these in your daily life? Use the following table to help plan the changes:

Cognitive defusion strategy	What situations could you plan to use this? How might it help?	What will you do? How will you remember to make the change?
Find an ARC to bridge difficult experiences		
Find the big picture perspective		
Scroll past like on social media		
Bad weather thoughts		
Thoughts on a TV screen		
Change the voice		
Write it out		
"I'm having the thought that…"		

4.7 Wise choices

We can use **Wise Mind** to help decide how to respond to difficult situations, thoughts and feelings. We may not be able to guarantee a specific outcome, but we can choose how to approach problems: whether to walk away, to talk to someone, what words to use, whether to pause and breathe, take a sip of a drink, read a book, or study for an exam. We have many choices and make many of these without even realising that we are doing so.

It's sometimes useful to think about **Wise Mind** as a bridge helping you over a turbulent river. The river is composed of all the negative and distressing thoughts, feelings, urges and memories that arise in a challenging situation. Using the bridge allows you to make Wise choices and take Wise actions to cross over towards what you care about. The bridge is the point at which there is **choice**.

Simply being aware that this choice exists can start to free us from feeling trapped by challenging life circumstances. Choosing actions that take us towards our values is likely to lead to increased wellbeing and a greater sense of meaning and satisfaction in life.

Is this helpful?

One of the key questions that **Wise Mind** asks about thoughts you choose to listen to, emotions that are driving your reactions and every action that you choose to take is: '**How helpful is this for me?**'

Your inner **Guide** can help answer this question. For each action you take, you can ask yourself: Is this action moving TOWARDS or AWAY from my values and the things that matter?

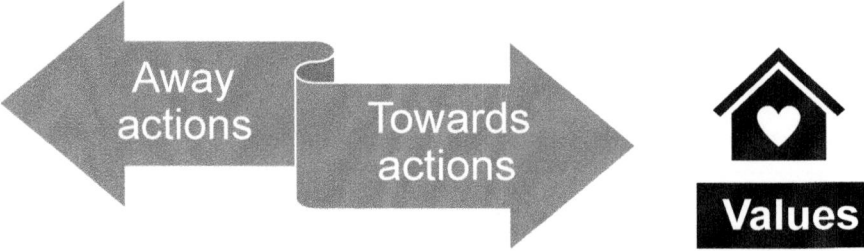

 PAUSE AND REFLECT: When facing a challenge or difficult situation, pause and ask yourself:

What am I thinking and feeling right now?	
If I let this thought, mindset or urge direct my behaviour, which direction will it take me in? Does it help me to be the person I want to be and do the things I want to do?	
Which value or need is important? Where is my inner **Guide** pointing?	
What advice can my **Wise Mind** offer in this situation?	

Neelam could take a moment to pause and notice her choices when she is feeling stressed and irritable with colleagues or her husband, or when she feels the urge to comfort eat or have another glass of wine.

She can engage with the present moment, using **Open and Observe** skills to recognise that she has feelings of irritability, and is experiencing worries about things going wrong, and has a sense of blame for others as well as herself.

She might pause and take a few slow exhales whilst acknowledging that this is a stressful and distressing moment. Then she can expand her perspective, using ARC to: **A**cknowledge her thoughts and feelings, **R**ecognise the urge to react and then notice that she has a **C**hoice and can use **Wise Mind** to help her make decisions about how to respond to difficult experiences.

"I could slip into automatic pilot and end up snapping at my husband or just reaching for the biscuit tin... or I could try to pause and notice how I'm feeling. I can recognise that even though this feels really uncomfortable, I do have a choice with how to respond. I can pick a Wise Action, so I might hold in the snappy comment and instead share with my colleague that I'm feeling stressed and ask for help. Or I might have a healthy snack or a drink of water or go for a walk, instead of automatically reaching for a cake or a glass of wine. It's helpful to remember that I can choose, and I don't have to fall into the same old patterns every time."

4.8 Support and encouragement

As clinicians, we often use **Wise Mind** to support our patients and colleagues. We can use this same supportive mindset when we relate to ourselves. This is like acting as a supportive mentor who helps you to find new ways to do things that lead to improvements in your life. You can act like a supportive coach who motivates through encouragement, kindness and wisdom, and has your best interests at heart, rather than through blame, shaming or constant criticism.

Have you come across an encouraging instructor, teacher, boss, friend or mentor at some point in your life? What qualities did they have? What would they say to you or to others who were struggling? How did they support or motivate you? Can you keep any of these qualities or advice in mind when facing difficulties in your own life?

We will talk more about the importance of offering ourselves self-compassion in *Chapter 5*. For now, if you notice that you are slipping into unhelpful thinking patterns such as self-criticism or blame, try using the following questions to bring to mind an encouraging inner supporter:

PAUSE AND REFLECT: Finding my inner mentor

What would I say to someone else who was struggling with this situation? How would I support a colleague or a friend?	
What wider perspective or context is relevant or important to take into account?	
What might a supportive coach or mentor say?	
How can I encourage myself without slipping into criticism or blame?	
What Wise choices can I make that follow my inner Guide and move me towards my values?	

Matthew comments: *"I am definitely my own biggest critic, and this can make it difficult to get my work done. I would never be so negative or tough on one of my friends or colleagues! It doesn't come very naturally, but I can see the benefit of being a bit more positive and encouraging. I had a really supportive football coach when I used to play regularly. She didn't ignore it when I had a difficult game but would always remind me of all the games that I had played well in the past and encourage me to think about what to try next time so I could improve my performance. If she was sitting next to me now, she would want me to do my best and to put in as much effort as I can, and she would also understand that I'm still learning and that I can't get things 100% right every time."*

4.9 Repetitive and intrusive thoughts

It's completely normal to experience repetitive thoughts. We have around 60,000 thoughts per day, and most of these are repeated multiple times over each day or week. It's only if we pay excessive attention to repetitive thoughts or allow them to distract us from carrying out our daily activities, that they can start to become a problem. If this happens, they can magnify in importance, trigger distressing emotions and unhelpful behaviours, and become a hindrance to enjoying our daily lives.

Let's look at some strategies for dealing with intrusive thoughts such as worry and rumination.

'Mind worms' and 'rapid relief'

Intrusive thoughts often involve repetitive inner conversations which spiral round in your mind. When you get excessively preoccupied and over-focused on these negative thoughts, we call this getting stuck with a 'mind worm'. This might involve worry, where you get stuck with repetitive thoughts about things that might go wrong. Other mind worms can involve repeated self-critical recriminations and blame about past events.

Mind worm: *"What if I freeze and forget my speech or can't read my slides in the presentation? It will be a disaster! I will be discredited....and look like a complete fool! Remember that time last year when I tripped over my words while I was presenting my audit in front of the whole team? I looked a total idiot and lost everyone's respect. I bet that happens again..."*

Our mind's natural response is often to try to find some comfort or a quick way out of the situation. This usually involves seeking reassurance or attempting to avoid the emotion or situation. We can call this **'rapid relief'**.

Rapid relief: *"Yes this is a very scary situation. How can I help you feel better? Come on, everything will be fine. You have done presentations before. I'm sure it wasn't really that bad last year, don't get so worked up! Why not just do lots more preparation… or have a drink beforehand? Or you could ask a colleague whether they think you are up to doing the task, I'm sure they would say that you will do well. If things get really bad, you can always call in sick!"*

Rapid relief strategies, such as seeking reassurance, avoidance, over-preparing, and trying to make absolutely certain, may ease the sting of the emotion and provide some short-term respite. But how long is it until the intrusive thoughts and the difficult emotions come back?

Rapid relief is trying to **rid** you of the problem, thought or emotion. But this is impossible, and it takes more effort in the long term because it is like feeding a hungry monster – the more you give it, the more it wants. So, you just keep spiralling around the same old path, bouncing backwards and forwards between the mind worm and rapid relief.

PAUSE AND REFLECT: Are you familiar with any of these common rapid relief strategies?

- Seeking reassurance
- Avoidance, escape or procrastination
- Seeking certainty and checking
- Perfectionism and unrealistic standards
- Over-preparing
- Trying to control, push away, eradicate or blot out difficult thoughts and feelings using behaviours such as alcohol, food or over-working.

A wise alternative

Cultivating our **Wise Mind** creates a quiet inner voice which acts as an alternative to the exhausting back and forth between mind worms and rapid relief. **Wise Mind** is thoughtful, reliable and dependable when we are struggling with difficult emotions. It is sometimes slower to come forward because it is responsive, using the 'high road' pathways of the brain, rather than the rapid stress pathways of the 'low road', but leads to a longer-term reduction in the frequency, intensity and distress associated with negative thoughts and feelings.

Wise Mind reviews the options and *chooses* how to respond. It is the voice of reason that steps back, acknowledges what is happening, investigates with a sense of kindness and curiosity and makes thoughtful choices that are in line with your personal values.

Wise Mind is like a thoughtful, diplomatic and caring leader of a team of complex characters, all with strong opinions and ideas. **Wise Mind** is accepting and allows all the different mindsets and thought patterns to be part of the team. It's like working with a collaborative mentor who respects everyone's view, but without colluding with them, arguing, or rejecting them, and without trying to take control through force or criticism.

Wise Mind does not treat thoughts and feelings as a threat, but as a guest. It recognises that feeling anxious is not the same as being in danger. Thoughts are not facts and thinking something does not make it happen. Being true to this wisdom allows us to diminish the importance of the thoughts and decreases the fear.

Wise Mind: *"Ah, here it is again! I can **observe** that I'm having thoughts about the presentation not going well. I can notice feelings of anxiety, and there is a sense of tightness in my chest and throat. I'm familiar with these sensations – they often arise when I want to do well or when I am excited or passionate about something. I'm going to be gentle with myself, pause and breathe with the thoughts and feelings for a moment, not trying to get rid of them and just accepting how I am feeling at this moment. Now I can notice that there are more confident thoughts coming up as well. I know I can do this well enough. I will focus on doing a bit of final preparation that will help it run more smoothly, and then go out for some fresh air and exercise."*

So, with **Wise Mind**, we might draw on some of the following:

- Recognition and acknowledgement of our inner experiences
- Willingness to take actions that move us towards our values even in the face of discomfort or distress
- Tolerance and acceptance of uncertainty and doubt
- Relaxing extreme standards – good enough is enough

- Know when you are prepared enough and then stop

- Responding with kindness and self-compassion.

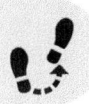

TAKE ACTION: Bring your Wise Mind to life

Choose a situation that you often find challenging, and in which you find a 'Mind Worm' can often capture your attention and keep you stuck in negative patterns of thinking or behaviour. How can you use your **Wise Mind** as an alternative to seeking rapid relief? What Wise actions can you commit to that might help you to step out of the cycle and improve your wellbeing?

Chapter summary: Wise Mind

- **Wise Mind** involves thinking flexibly and adapting our perspective to meet challenges and resolve difficulties.

- Noticing unhelpful thought patterns without struggling to get rid of them can help us to step back and choose how to respond in a helpful way.

- We can make Wise choices about which thoughts to listen to, how to react, and what action to take.

- **Wise Mind** helps us use an ARC as a bridge across discomfort and to find a big picture perspective that acts as an alternative to negative thinking.

- It may take the voice of a supportive coach or mentor, who motivates us through kindness and encouragement and keeps our best interests in mind.

- We can respond to intrusive thoughts using **Wise Mind** rather than rapid relief such as avoidance or seeking reassurance, which often worsens emotional distress in the long term.

Final thoughts

What are the most important messages for you from this chapter?

Take an action step

What are your next steps? What actions will you take as a result of reading this chapter?

How might you allow your **Wise Mind** to take a leadership role when making decisions, plans or responding to challenges?

05 Thrive and balance

- Do you feel emotionally balanced, energised and able to operate at your optimum level?

- Can you keep stress in check, or do you feel overwhelmed by juggling your workload with other pressures and responsibilities?

- Do you have enough time to wind down and recuperate, or are you on a treadmill of constant demands with a never ending to-do list?

- Let's look at ways to create balance and thrive in our daily lives...

5.1 The impact of stress

Stress is a modern reality that affects us all, both mentally and physically. It involves a range of neurochemical reactions including adrenaline, cortisol, serotonin and dopamine. In the introduction, we looked at some of the many causes of stress from working in primary care, including working long hours at high intensity, coping with unrealistic expectations and high levels of demand, dealing with uncertainty, the emotional toll of supporting patients who are distressed or suffering, fear of making mistakes, and professional isolation.

One important way of managing stress is to create a balance between the demands of work and those of other important aspects of our daily lives. Finding ways to recover mentally and physically from the challenges of work can also help to maximise wellbeing and performance.

In this chapter we will look at:

- Understanding our personal stress response

- Problem-solving ways to cope with stress triggers

- Using a 'three circles model' to help balance our different emotional systems

- Developing self-compassion to cope with challenging situations.

Let's look back at some of the previous healthcare staff who were coping with stress:

Inger, Salaried GP: *"I've found myself getting increasingly drained from the demands of my patients. By the end of the day, I'm exhausted and I'm starting to lose my empathy. I'm feeling increasingly tired and I'm just getting really overwhelmed especially during a long and busy day."*

Anna, Practice Pharmacist: *"I get really bogged down with all my work tasks, so I constantly leave late. At home I'm arguing with my partner because we hardly spend any time together in the evenings and I blame him for not doing more at home, even though he too works hard."*

Aftab, Nurse Practitioner: *"I had to gather patient and colleague feedback. Nearly all of it was positive, but there was a negative comment from one patient. Despite all the praise, all I could think about afterwards was this one negative comment that completely knocked my confidence."*

We will come back to these examples later in the chapter to explore ways to help each individual manage stress and improve their mental health and wellbeing.

5.2 What is stress?

We experience stress in situations or relationships where we see ourselves as lacking the personal skills, capabilities or resources to cope with the challenges that we are facing. The greater the demands of the situation, the higher our level of stress. Stressors may be internal or external and include feeling pressure to achieve a certain standard, manage relationships, meet social expectations, perform in front of others, or cope with time pressures.

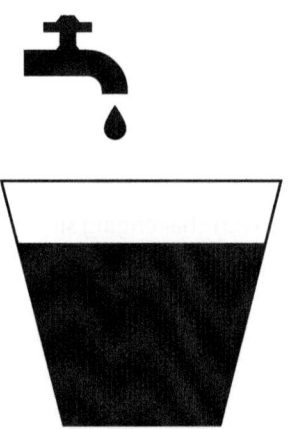

A 'stress bucket'

One helpful way to visualise stress is to imagine your 'stress bucket' (Brabban & Turkington, 2002). We can think of the demands and pressures in our lives as water being poured into a bucket. Over time, the water level, and our stress, will rise. The size of your bucket – how much stress you can personally hold without it flowing over – is influenced by your background, life experiences, personality traits and beliefs.

There are three ways to prevent the stress bucket from overflowing:

- Reduce the flow into the bucket by looking for ways to lessen pressures and demands

- Improve how well we drain the bucket by developing coping strategies for dealing with stress

- Increase the size or flexibility of the bucket by introducing self-compassion and finding support.

PAUSE AND REFLECT: Your stress bucket

What size and shape is your stress bucket? How full is it at the moment?	
What are the signs that your personal stress bucket is getting too full?	
What can you do to reduce the flow of stress into your bucket?	
What strategies do you turn to, to release stress? Are these healthy or unhealthy ways of coping under pressure?	

5.3 Factors influencing stress

Let's start by thinking about what stressors are contributing to your rising stress levels. These include external factors such as major life events, or the pressure of daily tasks. Helpful factors, such as a good support system or team spirit at work, can act to mitigate some of the demands.

Internal factors such as our personality, beliefs and habits may also make health professionals more prone to stress, and we look at these in *Chapter 7*.

PAUSE AND REFLECT: Triggers for stress

Let's explore some of the factors involved in triggering, increasing or maintaining stress in your life:

Factors influencing stress	Examples in your life
Major life events such as moving house, a bereavement, planning a big event, having a baby, or taking on a new role	
Practical difficulties such as a long commute, balancing work with childcare or other caring roles, and environmental factors such as noise, interruptions or inadequate working conditions	
Demands of work such as the quantity or intensity of work, deadlines, time pressures, demanding patients, targets, lack of stimulation, or not having necessary skills to cope with the challenges of the role	
Support at work, including management, supervision or feedback processes, peer support, teamwork, effective leadership, meetings, and the impact of protocols and organisational policies on your working role	
Autonomy – how much control you have over your work, and whether you can influence or implement outcomes or changes; whether you feel heard and are able to express your opinions and needs	
Wider life stresses and challenges that may impact on work or influence your overall reserves to cope with work-related demands and pressures	

Let's turn to our previous example of Inger, a Salaried GP who has been experiencing stress and overwhelm from the demands of her busy workload. She completes the table for her stress triggers:

Factors influencing stress	Inger's examples
Major life events	We are trying to sell our house and the sale has been really long and drawn-out due to problems with the buyer, and that's been very stressful.
Practical difficulties	My commute is currently about 45 minutes, which is quite long. I feel tense every day about finishing on time to pick up my son from nursery, and then with traffic we often get home late.
Demands of work	Work is busy and intense. There are frequent interruptions with people knocking on my door and asking me to do something. I find it hard to switch off and often find myself checking work emails and thinking about work on my day off.
Support at work	My practice manager is supportive, and I really like working with the GPs and nurses in the practice. Working part-time means I sometimes miss meetings, and I can feel isolated and be the last to find out when something has changed.
Autonomy	I don't feel the partners really understand my perspective. Nothing seems to change, even when I point out problems at the practice and suggest solutions.
Wider life stresses and challenges	My mother has been poorly and has been into hospital recently. I'm worried that she may need surgery. She needs support during outpatient appointments, and I feel guilty that I can rarely attend with her.

5.4 Stress, pressure and performance

It's helpful to make a distinction between stress and pressure. A reasonable level of pressure can help us to respond to the challenges of daily life, keeping us energised and alert, and motivating us to keep going through challenging situations. Noticing when pressure is moving towards stress and becoming less healthy can act as a warning sign that reminds us to take time out or make changes to our lives. One way to understand stress and pressure is to look at different performance zones:

Performance zone	Level of pressure	Characteristics of this zone
Comfort zone	Low pressure / low achievement	The comfort zone feels safe and secure, with few challenges. It is perfect for resting and relaxing. Getting stuck in a rut in the comfort zone may restrict your life and can lead to stagnation and boredom. Constantly avoiding challenges may also have a negative impact on confidence.
Stretch zone	Low to moderate pressure and achievement	As you take on more challenges, there is an increase in pressure and a greater sense of accomplishment. Staying in this zone involves coping with obstacles and finding new pathways to successful outcomes. Support and collaboration with colleagues and leaders will help you to function effectively in this zone.
High-performance zone	Moderate to high pressure and achievement	This is a zone of maximum performance and exceptional achievement where meeting challenging goals offers an immense sense of satisfaction. However, spending too long in the upper end of this zone without rest and recuperation is exhausting and may eventually lead to a depletion in your reserves.
Overload zone	High stress and lower achievement	Pressure has become excessive and created high levels of stress. You become fatigued, and your performance, confidence and decision-making deteriorate, with a risk of burnout. It's better to avoid reaching overload, but you can also use it as a signal to actively seek ways to move back to a lower zone. It's not necessary to retreat all the way back to the comfort zone, but occasionally this might provide a short respite that re-energises you to then move back up into the zones of optimal performance.

5.5 Coping with stress

If we recognise pressure and stress early, we have an opportunity to take action! There are two main strategies for coping with stress: problem-solving and learning to manage stress emotions.

Problem-solving to reduce stress

This is a practical approach which involves trying to change the situations or triggers for stress. This is most helpful when we have some autonomy or ability to alter the circumstances causing stress, and for problems that can change or have potential solutions. It's also helpful to identify small stress triggers that might be easier to resolve.

Let's turn back to Inger and her list of stress triggers. She goes back through the list and picks some important examples. The next step is to brainstorm any solutions or coping strategies that might help her to manage the problem more effectively.

Factors influencing stress	Pinpoint the problem and list possible solutions or coping strategies	What are the first steps?
Delays in selling our house	I've been avoiding the paperwork for the move because I feel anxious thinking about it. Completing this would make me feel more in control and less stressed	Make a list of the documents that need to be completed Plan a time to fill these in next weekend with my husband.
Long commute	Having food already prepared when we get home would help me manage the evening routine I also get tense and irritable when there is traffic on the journey home. I could try to use this as wind-down time instead, using audiobooks in the car	Cook and freeze an extra portion of food on my day off Occasionally have sandwiches or a cold meal at dinner time Buy some audiobooks
Stresses and demands at work	I am constantly interrupted by requests from others. Reducing these would help me be more efficient at work It's hard to switch off after work, but it would be helpful to keep a boundary between work and family life	Remove my work email from my phone so I can't check at home Ask my team to avoid interruptions unless I'm the duty doctor Say 'no' more often to things that aren't my responsibility, or ask for support
Support at work	Staying isolated in my room means I miss out on the company of colleagues and catching up on information	Make sure I leave my room for a coffee break at least 3 times a week Have lunch with a colleague rather than at my desk
My mother's illness	My family often turn to me as the only doctor, but I have two brothers who could be more involved	Phone my older brother and discuss how we can support mum as a family, and whether he could go to any appointments with her

Now look back at your own answers to the exercise on factors influencing stress. Try to pick out any practical problems that are likely to have realistic solutions. Can you reduce demands, increase coping strategies or seek support? List things that you could try, and use these to complete the following table:

Factors influencing stress	Pinpoint the problem and list solutions or coping strategies	What are the first steps?

We will look further at ways to cope with challenging and stressful life experiences in *Chapter 11* on surviving significant events.

Coping with stress emotions

It's also important to find ways to cope with our stress emotions, especially when some stress triggers are difficult to eliminate, or are outside our control. In the next section, we will look at ways to understand and manage our stress emotions using a three circles model.

5.6 Three circles model of emotions

The three circles model of emotions (see figure below) helps explain how the body and mind respond to stress, by looking at the relationship between three different emotional systems (Gilbert, 2010):

- Threat system

- Drive system

- Calm and connect system.

Each has an important role to play in managing our physical and mental health. Creating a balance between the systems can help to maximise our performance and wellbeing.

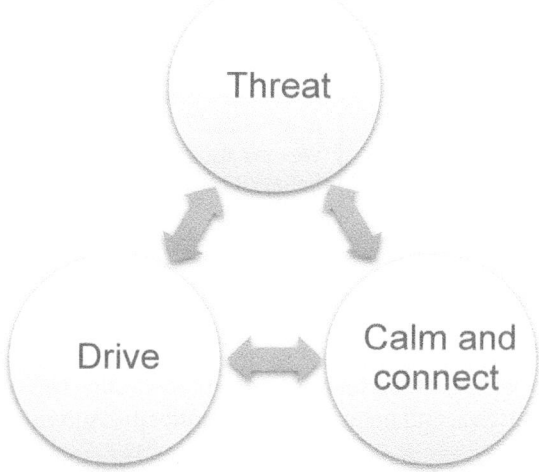

Threat system

When we encounter a stressful or threatening situation, the threat system activates our basic survival response. This could be an external threat, such as dealing with an abusive or angry patient in the waiting room, or coping with mounting emails, results and deadlines. Other threats may be internal, arising from thoughts and beliefs, such as worrying about possible future difficulties, or attacking ourselves with harsh, self-critical thoughts.

Our brains respond to both external and internal threats, real or imagined, in exactly the same way. The threat system triggers the fight, flight or freeze reaction using the 'low road' pathways of the brain which we introduced in *Section 3.7*.

Overview of the threat system

How it evolved	For survival and self-protection
What it does	Alerts us to potential danger and motivates us to take action to stay safe by triggering the fight, flight or freeze response
Systems involved	Sympathetic nervous system triggers stress hormones, including adrenaline and cortisol
Thoughts and thinking styles	High alert and awareness of danger May trigger anxious, catastrophic and self-critical thoughts focusing on mistakes, problems and risk

Emotions	Fear, anger, disgust, embarrassment, shame and numbness
Physical reactions	Increased heart rate, muscle tension, and sharpened senses as we prepare to confront or run away from the danger Other physiological responses include sweating, shaking, rapid breathing and gastrointestinal changes
Behaviour	Aggression, defensiveness and escape; with severe threat, we may freeze We may also try to reduce the perception of risk using behaviour such as avoidance, checking, reassurance-seeking or numbing out

How does the threat system help us?

The threat system activates our brain and body to stay alert for potential dangers, and then take action to protect ourselves and stay safe. This is essential for survival and helps us to cope under pressure.

What problems can develop with the threat system?

The threat system is often the fastest system to activate and may be slower to settle down again. The 'negativity bias' of the brain means we often give priority to dealing with threats rather than enjoying pleasant things. And if we spend lots of time living in a state of threat, our lives become stressful, exhausting and overwhelming. It's also unhelpful if our threat system is activated when we are trying to connect with others or when we are lying in bed trying to relax or fall asleep.

The threat system is also less effective at coping with future problems that cannot be resolved in the here and now. It operates on a 'better safe than sorry' principle, meaning that our brains can overestimate, imagine and ruminate about many different threats and dangers, and the system can remain active even in the absence of any actual external threat.

Balancing the threat system

Balancing the threat system involves learning to cope with risk and uncertainty. This involves being able to recognise and taking reasonable steps to stay safe if there is real danger, but without resorting to unhelpful or repetitive safety behaviours which reduce our quality of life.

We can view the threat system as a highly sensitive alarm, rather than something to be eliminated. If a smoke alarm is set off by burnt toast, we don't throw the alarm in the bin! Instead, we check if there's a fire, and if not, turn it off and get on with our day.

Key skills for managing the threat system include:

- Use **Open and Observe** skills to recognise when the threat system is triggered. Pause and make space to step out of the automatic reaction and engage your high road pathways using exercises in *Chapter 3* such as 'notice the NOW' (see *Section 3.2*) and 'steady yourself with your five senses' (see *Section 3.8*).

- Gain perspective and choose to listen to **Wise Mind**, rather than catastrophic, worst-case predictions, or the urge to seek 'rapid relief' for uncomfortable feelings.

- Approach rather than avoid stressful situations in small, graded steps to build your confidence.

- Cut back on unhelpful behaviours that maintain the anxiety cycle, such as checking, reassurance-seeking, excessive alcohol or caffeine.

- Respond to pressure by stepping out of the threat circle and activating one of the other emotion systems such as drive or calm and connect.

We will look at more ways to respond to anxiety and worry in *Chapter 9*.

Anna, Pharmacist: *"I'm so tired and stressed with the volume of work and I'm afraid of making an error on a prescription. That makes me over-cautious and I'm checking more, which slows me up and makes me get home even later. It's keeping me awake at night and I'm starting to get palpitations when I think of my workload. I'm thinking of looking for a change of career, even though I used to love my job and I know I can do it well."*

PAUSE AND REFLECT: An overactive threat system

What signs do you notice that Anna's threat system is overactive?

Let's now review how Anna could apply some of the skills that we have covered so far to balance threat:

Anna's reflections:

I know my threat system is over-active because I constantly feel tense, stressed, edgy and irritable.

- *Inner Guide: Professional satisfaction is important to me; I want to enjoy and feel pride in my job. I also want to be able to relax and enjoy time away from work.*

- **Ready for Action**: I could try to break down my tasks into more manageable steps, so I don't feel so overwhelmed. And when I've completed some prescriptions, I will immediately pass them on to the admin team, so I'm less tempted to constantly double-check.

- **Open and Observe**: I could notice and name how I am thinking and feeling or try listening to a short mindfulness track when I get home from work to help let go of any worries. It might also help to go for a walk with the dog before talking to my husband! At work I will try to notice the NOW if I'm getting anxious.

- **Wise mind**: Looking at the bigger picture, my balanced perspective is that I'm good at my job and I've always enjoyed it. It would be a shame to lose that because of anxiety. If I can rebuild my confidence and step out of the threat circle a bit more, I think I would feel much happier.

Drive system

Drive is a motivational system which helps us to get things done. Activating drive involves pursuing, striving and achieving, as we seek out what we need to survive and prosper. Each time we pass an exam, get a promotion, win a competition, or achieve any goal that we have set for ourselves, we engage the drive system.

Overview of the drive system

How it evolved	To motivate us to seek out the things we want or need in life
What it does	Creates positive emotions and builds a sense of self-esteem when we experience success
Systems involved	The release of dopamine by the brain produces a rush of excitement or pleasure when we achieve our goals
Typical emotions	We experience feelings of joy, fun, excitement and pleasure with every success. If our desires and goals are blocked, we may perceive this as a threat, leading to anxiety, frustration or anger.
Physical reactions	There is often a 'buzz' or 'rush' of excitement which can be addictive and lead to overuse of the drive system. In 'over-drive', we become over-stimulated, with sleep problems, a racing mind, and difficulty relaxing or winding down. Persistent over- or under-use of the drive system can cause fatigue and exhaustion.
Behaviour	The drive system helps us concentrate on actions that lead towards important goals. However, if we overuse this system, we may become obsessional and over-focused on specific goals or targets. It can also lead to addictive or thrill-seeking behaviour.

How does the drive system help?

When in balance with the other emotional systems, drive helps us to build positive relationships and self-esteem. Drive is often a superpower for many health professionals, who are typically high achievers and extremely successful in many areas of life. We are experts at working hard and achieving our goals. And this is a highly functional and useful life skill… without it we would never get anything done!

What problems can develop with the drive system?

If we get stuck in 'over-drive' we may focus on work to the detriment of other aspects of our lives, and without allowing time to rest and recuperate. We may get addicted to achievement, constantly seeking success in unrelenting, obsessional ways. This can lead to overwork, stress, perfectionism and burnout, or addictive and compulsive behaviours such as alcohol or substance abuse, gambling or extreme risk activities.

In burnout or low mood, we may get stuck in 'under-drive'. Here we become demotivated and lose confidence, so we cut back on our usual activities and lose the sense of achievement from regularly activating our drive system. We cover this more in *Chapter 8*.

Threat and drive

When used wisely, drive can be a helpful system for managing threat. When stressed and busy, we can use drive to motivate us to face difficulties, find solutions, and feel good about our achievements.

However, we may also overuse the drive system, causing increased stress and pressure to achieve as we constantly bounce between threat and drive in a never-ending spiral. And 'failing' to achieve goals, no matter how challenging or unrealistic they may be, can lead to punishing self-criticism and feelings of shame. We may also get pulled into less healthy ways of managing the sense of threat, such as alcohol or substance misuse.

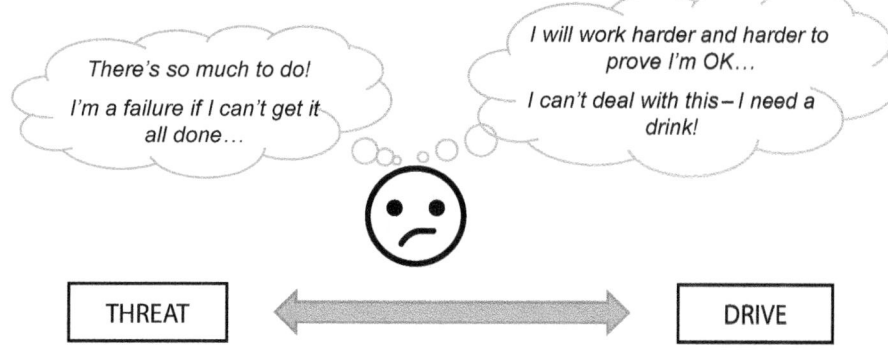

Mo, GP Trainee: *"I am passionate about my work and want to do well. I have ambition to become a Partner as soon as possible and influence decisions in the practice. I often stay late at work, and then study when I get home. I also enjoy running and I'm entering some local athletics championships. I get frustrated if I don't feel I've done well enough and find myself constantly striving to do better which can be exhausting. My fiancée says I'm neglecting her as she is not sporty and prefers gentle walks to running. She says I am never satisfied and it's affecting our relationship. Maybe I need to re-think things..."*

PAUSE AND REFLECT: Balancing threat and drive

- Is Mo following his inner **Guide**? What important values is he neglecting?

- What internal demands are sending Mo's system into over-drive?

- Can you recognise any similarities? Make a note of your thoughts:

Balancing the drive system

The first step is to recognise how much time and energy you are putting into your drive system:

- Are you over-working? Is the drive to achieve goals getting in the way of enjoying life and connecting with others?

- Are you using achievement, alcohol or extreme activities to cope with difficult feelings?

- Are you demotivated and lacking a sense of achievement or purpose?

Here are some simple steps for balancing the drive system:

- Use your inner **Guide**. Notice how much time you are spending each day focusing on goals and achievements. Goals are important but are not sufficient for wellbeing if you are not taking time to rest or connect with friends and family.

- Broaden your definition of achievement to include a more balanced range of activities that connect with your values.

- Plan actions which are realistic and achievable. In over-drive, try setting participation goals rather than outcome-based goals, such as "I will engage regularly in physical activity over the week" rather than "I need to run at least 10km". This allows greater flexibility to match our planned activities to changing priorities and time pressures, rather than seeing ourselves as 'failing' to achieve unrealistic standards.

- If you are struggling with motivation, try planning very small steps that are connected to your most important values, such as self-care, professionalism and relationships with others. We talk more about this in *Chapter 7* on low mood.

Mo reflects: "*I do get a real kick out of all the things that I achieve in life, but I can see that my drive system has got a bit out of control. It's become quite demanding, and I no longer get so much enjoyment – I feel pressurised and stressed and constantly feel that I'm failing to do enough. I can see that it would help to be more realistic about my expectations of myself. I don't have to compete in athletics – I enjoy being active but not at the expense of my relationships. I will start planning some nature walks with my fiancée and some other activities we can enjoy together.*"

Calm and connect system

The calm and connect system is essential for helping us to switch off and recover but is often underused when we are busy or under stress. When there are no threats to defend against and no goals that must be pursued, it enables us to feel safe, calm, peaceful and content. We soothe ourselves and connect with others as we give and receive affection, kindness, warmth and support.

Overview of the calm and connect system

How it evolved	To enable us to respond to emotional distress in ourselves and others. It is linked to the attachment system which encourages adult mammals to nurture and care for their vulnerable young offspring. It also motivates us to give and receive support from others, ensuring cooperation and connection.
What it does	It motivates us to nurture and care for ourselves and for others and allows us to rest and feel content. It also enables us to feel soothed in the presence of a caring person.
Systems involved	The parasympathetic nervous system and a variety of neurochemicals including oxytocin, endorphins and opiates

Typical emotions	Feelings of contentment, without striving or seeking to make change. There are also feelings of safety, connectedness, affection and kindness.
Physical reactions	Our bodies respond to closeness and touch from others by relaxing and lowering our heart rate. 'Coregulation' means that affection and kindness from others can help to calm us when we are distressed, and that we can soothe others.
Behaviour	It is linked with experiences of giving and receiving affection and care from others, including behaviour that demonstrates acceptance, kindness and support. This also includes showing kindness and compassion towards ourselves and creating space and time to nurture and meet our own needs.

How does the calm and connect system help?

The calm and connect system helps to down-regulate the threat response, allowing us to relax, feel peaceful and at ease. It also allows us to feel safe and connected to the people around us.

What problems can develop with the calm and connect system?

Underuse of the calm and connect system means that we may experience harsh, judgemental or self-critical thoughts, particularly when things go wrong. It's helpful to understand that this inner voice is trying to ensure that we avoid mistakes and live up to our potential. But, trying to motivate ourselves through criticism means that we can become demoralised and start to feel that we can never do or be enough.

Early attachment bonds with caregivers shape the development of the calm and connect system and contribute to our ability to regulate emotions. The experience of rejection, abuse, lack of empathy, or unresponsiveness from parents or carers can influence our relationships in adult life, including whether we perceive others as predictable or trustworthy, and how we care for ourselves during times of emotional distress.

Balancing the calm and connect system

Are you underusing your calm and connect system? Is it in balance with the other systems, or are you bouncing between threat and drive and risking emotional and physical exhaustion?

Some strategies for engaging the calm and connect system include:

- Seek out and spend time with people who make you feel warm, safe, happy and accepted. Acknowledge and recognise your needs for self-care, mutual support and wellbeing, and actively find ways to meet these in your daily life.

- Make time for calming activities such as taking a relaxing bath, a massage, doing a jigsaw, knitting, reading, painting or yoga.

- Recognise your need for care and calm. Use your five senses to connect with and appreciate nature or a calm environment, or practise mindfulness and gratitude. Stimulate the parasympathetic nervous system with slow exhalations, singing or relaxation. Use imagery, such as creating an image of a safe place, being wrapped in a warm, comforting blanket or having a compassionate or caring companion to support you.

- Listen to your wise inner coach rather than your inner critic and practise self-compassion. Smile and make friendly eye contact with others or bring your facial expression into a gentle or 'half' smile. Think about 'smiling on the inside.'

PAUSE AND REFLECT: Expanding your calm and connect system

If you have a tendency to underuse your calm and connect system, what small steps could you take that might start to bring it into balance with the other systems?

5.7 The role of self-compassion

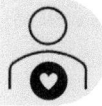

Self-compassion offers another way to engage the calm and connect system and is increasingly recognised as an essential component of wellbeing and self-care. It can help us to develop the resilience to cope with the stresses and challenges of caring for ourselves and others. And it is a skill that can be learnt and developed at any stage in life.

Self-compassion is particularly important when things go wrong. When we've made a mistake or are facing a complaint or a significant event, clinicians are particularly vulnerable to mental health difficulties. Self-compassion can help to balance the tendency to slip into self-criticism and blame, which triggers the threat system, and leads to powerful feelings of guilt and shame, particularly if we are conscientious or have perfectionist traits.

The self-compassion model acknowledges that the human brain sometimes creates a paradox: it has evolved to enable us to solve complex problems in the physical world, and this incredible ability allows us to function as competent and highly skilled professionals. However, this same problem-solving logic is less effective at dealing with emotional problems such as experiencing unwanted thoughts or feelings of stress and anxiety. In fact, our brains can worsen the distress by going into over-drive trying to resolve impossible dilemmas and triggering the threat system with self-criticism and blame for struggling to cope.

What is self-compassion?

Self-compassion involves a range of different qualities. Many health professionals demonstrate a huge capacity for care for others but may struggle to draw on this when facing their own difficulties.

Some important aspects of self-compassion include:

- Giving ourselves the same kindness, diplomacy and understanding that we would offer to friends, colleagues and peers, rather than slipping into self-criticism or judgement.

- Recognising that we are not alone and that many others share our experiences and challenges.

- Self-acceptance and remembering that we are not super-human or indestructible, but simply imperfect beings doing our best to cope with life's challenges.

- Setting realistic, fair expectations rather than perfectionist demands.

- Seeing difficulties and problems as an inevitable part of life, rather than indicating a deep personal flaw.

- Looking for ways to cope with mistakes rather than criticising, blaming or 'kicking ourselves when we are down'.

- Using mindful awareness to keep a balanced and non-judgemental perspective on painful or distressing thoughts and feelings.

- Maintaining a balanced perspective that keeps in mind positive as well as negative experiences.

- Seeking out and using support and care from others when needed.

PAUSE AND REFLECT: Experiencing compassion

Complete the following table to reflect on recent examples when you have experienced giving and receiving compassion:

Choose an example of...	Where were you? What did you do and say?	How did you feel: body and emotions?	What was the outcome?
A recent time that you have shown kindness or compassion to another person at work – a colleague or a patient			
A time when you have shown less compassion, or reacted with anger, irritation or impatience, towards a colleague, patient, family member or friend			
An experience where you were given compassion, care or support from someone else			

Now ask yourself:

- What do you notice from these examples?
- What are the benefits of compassion?
- Are there any challenges or difficulties with giving or receiving compassion?
- Can you think of any ways to increase your compassion to yourself and others?

Compassion through action

Compassion is more than an attitude or mindset; it also involves actions and behaviour. We can express self-compassion in action by actively looking for ways to show ourselves care. This involves prioritising our wellbeing through our choice of daily actions, and not letting this get squeezed out because we are too busy to look after ourselves.

Self-compassion in action might look like finding 10 minutes to read a book, do some drawing or yoga, take a restful bath, or spend time with people we care about. It might also involve 'standing tall', setting boundaries, and prioritising our own needs alongside those of other people.

PAUSE AND REFLECT: Bringing compassion to life

How might you bring compassion through action into your life? What steps could you plan that demonstrate your care for yourself? Can you reach out and connect to someone supportive? Can you commit to one or more micro-steps towards self-compassion in the next few days or weeks?

5.8 Developing self-compassion

Developing compassion for ourselves and others not only reduces personal emotional distress but also helps build relationships with colleagues and in our personal lives. Here are some strategies for developing different aspects of self-compassion:

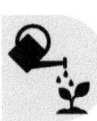

Aspect of self-compassion	What it involves	How can we develop this?
Care and nurture	Being able to offer ourselves support, encouragement, acceptance and nurture	Notice your inner critic and remind yourself that no one can be perfect. Try to stop punishing yourself for mistakes. Put a sticky note near your desk or a friendly reminder on your phone to be kind to yourself when you need it. Try a mindful self-compassion practice. There are many free apps and websites available.

| | Wisdom and perspective | Developing your ability to draw on experience and understanding, and seeing the big picture
Making choices about how to look after yourself and cope with life's inevitable difficulties | Use a diary to keep a reminder of successes and things that went well, to motivate you to keep going when facing problems and to counter any negative bias.
Develop a sense of gratitude and appreciation: try completing a daily journal, reflecting at bedtime, or taking a 'gratitude walk'.
Imagine looking down at the world from a high mountain or a tall building. What does life look like from up here? How might this help you gain perspective on any problems you are facing? |
| | Standing tall | Recognising your needs and noticing when situations or others do not embrace respect, equality and care | Voice your feelings and needs calmly and clearly, embracing equality and making reasonable requests of others.
Set boundaries and say no when needed.
Take a stand against discrimination or injustice. |

PAUSE AND REFLECT: Cultivating self-compassion

How might you start to cultivate the different aspects of self-compassion? Make a list of ideas in the table below:

Aspect of self-compassion	How could this help me?	What actions can I take to develop this?
Care and nurture		
Wisdom and perspective		
Standing tall		

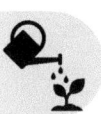

Aftab, Nurse Practitioner: *"I found it really hard to get a negative comment from a patient out of my mind, even though there was lots of praise from everyone else. When I got home, I felt so upset, I shouted at my son for not doing his homework properly. I don't want to be a demanding parent – I've always tried to be supportive and loving. After that I felt even worse, like I was failing in every way possible."*

PAUSE AND REFLECT: Coping with a difficult patient interaction

Think about the different aspects of self-compassion. How might Aftab:

- Give himself some self-care or nurture whilst following his **Guide**?
- Use **Wise Mind** and gain perspective when reflecting and making decisions?
- Stand tall and embrace his own needs and those of others around him?

Do you recognise any similarities? Do you ever slip into self-criticism when things go wrong? Make a note of your thoughts here:

Aftab's thoughts: *I can see that I was being quite tough on myself. I was ignoring all the positive feedback and just focusing on one small negative. I don't want to let that get in the way of my relationship with my son.*

I took a deep breath and read back through all the positive comments from the other patients. Then I spoke to a colleague who I respect. She helped me get some perspective as we laughed about some of the funny complaints we've both had over the years from patients. It's not possible to please everyone all the time, but I am doing my best.

I decided to be kind to myself and buy a nice sandwich for lunch. I took time to get a break and sat on a bench outside to eat it, enjoying the sunshine and the fresh air. When I got home, I had a relaxing shower and afterwards said sorry to my son for snapping the day before. I acknowledged his effort in attempting his homework and asked how things were going. He was surprisingly understanding! We went for a walk together and it was good to hear about his day.

5.9 Balancing the circles

Seeking wellbeing and managing stress involves finding a balance between the three systems. Think back over the past few days or weeks and answer the following questions:

EXERCISE: Your three circles

How much time or energy are you spending in each system: Threat, Drive, and Calm and connect?

Draw your own version of the three circles model showing how big, heavy or 'hot' each of the circles are, or use the template below:

What actions are you taking in each circle?

Complete the circles below with examples of actions that you are taking in each system, for example:

- **Threat:** thinking a lot about work, checking emails on my days off, keeping work phone on at home

- **Drive:** prioritising work tasks, setting ambitious targets, aiming to run a marathon, over-committed to tasks in personal and work life

- **Calm and connect:** taking time to chat to my partner or friends about my day, switching off by taking a bath, reading to my children, stroking the cat, appreciating my garden.

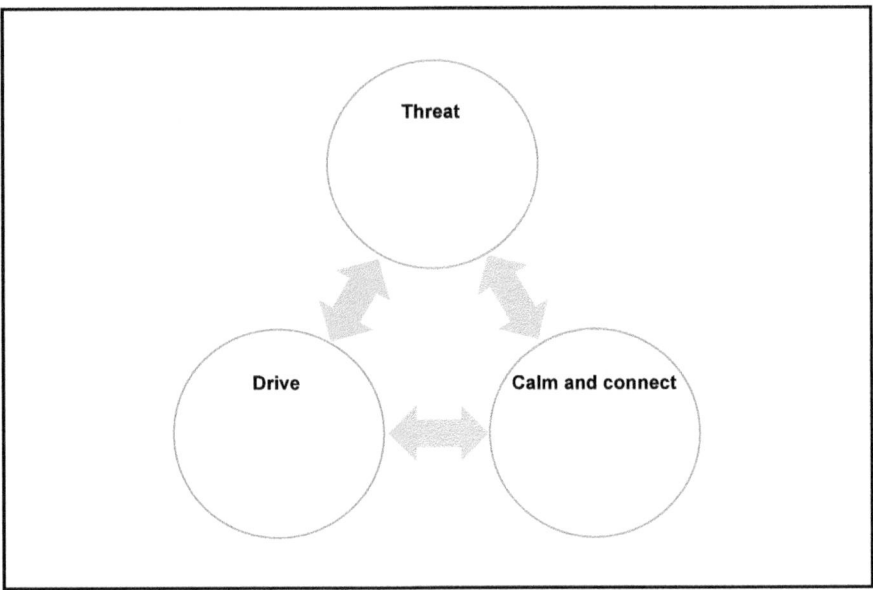

Chapter summary: Thrive and Balance

- Managing how much stress you experience can involve reducing demands and problem-solving practical solutions for stress triggers.

- Finding ways to thrive under pressure involves balancing the three emotion systems – Threat, Drive and Calm and Connect – as you:
    - Use your inner **Guide** and be **Ready for Action** by using the drive system wisely, choosing realistic small steps that move you towards your values
    - Be **Open and Observe** early warning signs that the threat system is triggered. Use your five senses to direct your attention away from excessive threat and engage with the present moment, resisting the urge to fall back on avoidance, reassurance and checking.
    - Use **Wise Mind** to listen to your compassionate inner voice rather than your anxious critic, and find small ways to show yourself care and connect with others.

Final thoughts

What are the most important messages for you from this chapter?

Take an action step

What are your next steps? What actions will you take as a result of reading this chapter?

What practical steps can you take to manage your stress and keep your emotion systems in balance?

06 Healthy Life Habits

- Do you know the theory of a healthy lifestyle, but feel too busy or stressed to apply it in practice?

- Do you have trouble sleeping, or unhealthy habits around nutrition, physical activity or social media?

- Do you keep procrastinating over taking action on your own health needs?

- Keep reading to create your own **Healthy Life Habits**…

6.1 What are Healthy Life Habits?

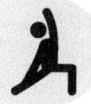

Building **Healthy Life Habits** can support our happiness and wellbeing, enabling us to meet a range of needs relating to physical, mental, emotional, spiritual, environmental and social health. In this chapter we will look at building healthy life habits, which includes:

- Being physically active

- Having healthy eating patterns and maintaining a healthy body weight

- Getting enough sleep

- Cutting back on unhealthy choices by, for example, not smoking, limiting alcohol intake and avoiding substance misuse

- Keeping unhealthy habits and addictive behaviours in check, such as excessive use of technology or 'hurry habits'

- Caring for your physical health, including managing long-term conditions and physical illness

- Strengthening relationships with important others. We look at this in *Chapter 10.*

6.2 What gets in the way?

As health professionals, we know the lifestyle behaviours that are good for physical and mental wellbeing, yet many of us still struggle to stick to healthy lifestyle choices. How easy do you find it to balance a healthy lifestyle with other priorities such as work, relationships and family commitments?

The key is to make lifestyle choices that suit you personally and focus on what's most important to you. This can motivate you to take action, encourage you to make wise choices, and help create a set of realistic habits that you can fit into your life. And we will look at ways to use the **GROWTH** steps to create repeatable **Healthy Life Habits** that are easy to maintain.

It's also important to make yourself a priority. You need to find a balance and a healthy routine that works for you, without pushing yourself too hard or setting unrealistic expectations for immediate results. This is a life journey! And it begins with one micro-step in the right direction.

Penny is a GP Partner and Trainer who works 7 sessions per week in her practice. She also has a family with two teenage daughters.

"I just don't seem to have time in my busy week to fit in all the things I know I should be doing to look after myself better. Over the years my weight has crept upwards, and since starting the menopause a few years ago I've found it really hard to keep it in check.

I don't enjoy exercise – I used to go to the gym regularly but I haven't been for over 6 months. I'm so busy with work and home-life – I never really seem to find the time. My daughters are my priority outside work and I always seem to be rushing to get them to their acitivities, leaving little time for myself.

I had a shock recently when I visited my own GP. My blood pressure was a bit high and a blood test found that I have pre-diabetes. My mum had diabetes and I suppose it's no surprise given my weight and lifestyle, but it felt like a real blow. I felt really bad and blamed myself for allowing this to happen.

I feel demotivated and I don't know where to start with making a change – it all feels too overwhelming."

PAUSE AND REFLECT: Where are you now?

Take a moment to pause and reflect on your current healthy life habits, and any challenges or areas that you might wish to change or improve:

Healthy life habits	What are you doing already that's helpful?	What are the challenges or difficulties? What would you wish to change or improve?
Physical activity Are you physically active during the day or mostly sedentary? How much moderate or vigorous exercise do you participate in regularly?		
Healthy eating and weight Do you have regular eating patterns and a balance of healthy nutrition that works for your body and lifestyle? Are you able to maintain a healthy weight?		
Sleep Do you have regular sleep patterns that meet your sleep requirements? How easy is it to drop off to sleep? How's the quality of your sleep?		
Unhealthy choices Do you engage in any unhealthy behaviours that may affect your health or wellbeing (e.g. smoking, drinking too much alcohol, other drugs)?		
Other unhealthy habits Do you have any other habits that might affect wellbeing, such as overuse of social media?		
Physical health Do you have any long-term health conditions or persistent physical symptoms which affect your wellbeing?		

 What have you learned from this exercise? What healthy life habits or areas would you like to work on?

6.3 Finding motivation to change

Thinking about your personal reasons for changing health behaviour can help overcome any ambivalence or uncertainty and motivate you to get started. This involves turning to your inner **Guide** and thinking about how **Healthy Life Habits** might move you towards your important values. This also involves thinking about the benefits and costs of changing versus those of not changing, as well as your willingness, ability and readiness to change.

PAUSE AND REFLECT: What are your reasons for healthy habits?

- What would encourage you to make the effort to change your health habits?
- What is important about it and what do you value most?
- Are you confident on what to change and how to do it?
- What are the costs and benefits of making a change?

6.4 Physical activity

The benefits of keeping active cannot be exaggerated. It has major benefits for emotional and physical health. Take a look at the chart below and reflect on what is most important to you:

Benefit of physical activity	Examples	How is this important to you personally?
Improves physical health	Reduced risk of cardiovascular disease, hypertension, diabetes and cancer. Boosts immunity, strengthens muscles and bones, reduces body fat, and helps maintain a healthy weight.	
Improves mood and reduces stress	Lifts low mood, increases energy, reduces stress, anxiety, irritability and depression, improves sleep.	
Social interaction	Creates opportunities to connect with others and brings shared meaning and purpose.	

Concentration and focus	Improves concentration, memory, focus and thinking skills. It can help improve efficiency at work and break up long periods of sitting in front of the computer.	
Develop self-confidence	Opportunities to learn or improve skills can build confidence and self-esteem.	

How much activity?

Adults are recommended to carry out at least 150 minutes of moderate or 75 minutes of vigorous physical activity or exercise per week, including both aerobic exercise and exercises for strength and balance. It's also important to minimise time spent being sedentary.

If you are already very committed to sport and activity, this may not sound like enough. Alternatively, if you work full-time, are juggling the needs of running a home and childcare, and have lost the habit of physical activity, this may seem impossible. The goal is to start from where you are now, rather than where you believe you 'should' be, and make small steps towards sustainable, realistic change.

What kind of exercise?

Different people enjoy different types of activity. One person might love organised team sports, whilst another may prefer non-competitive activities such as hiking or canoeing. It's important to look for physical activities that you enjoy, as well as bringing more physical movement into your daily routine.

Moderate to vigorous physical activity

During moderate activity, your heart rate starts to increase, and you will be breathing faster and feeling warmer. These activities can help to balance strong emotions, create feelings of happiness and wellbeing, and boost your energy. Examples include:

- Brisk walking or hiking

- Running, cycling, or swimming

- Circuit training or high intensity interval workouts

- Mowing the lawn or gardening

- Sports, such as golf, tennis, badminton, football or hockey

- Bouncing on a trampoline.

Strengthening activities

Activities that improve muscle or bone strength, balance and flexibility may provide an opportunity to connect socially and can also improve concentration and help settle a busy mind. They can also build self-esteem as we notice our achievements and feel positive about choosing to invest in our own wellbeing. Examples include:

- Yoga or Pilates
- Weights or gym workouts
- Martial arts
- Rock climbing
- Gymnastics
- Dance.

Reducing sedentary activity

How much time do you spend each day being inactive or sedentary? Activities such as sitting at a computer, travelling in a car, watching television or reading are part of modern life, but we need to balance them with other activities where we are active and moving. There are many ways to do this, such as:

- Setting an alarm to remind you to stand up and stretch your legs when working or sitting
- Investing in a standing desk
- Setting a goal for a daily number of steps using a pedometer
- Walking or cycling rather than taking a bus or car
- Keeping moving during your usual activities: go for a walk while talking on the phone, read an article when standing up, or listen to a podcast as you do chores at home or organise your workspace.

Getting moving

Here are some of our ideas for increasing your physical activity:

Physical activity habits	What could you try?
Schedule it in: Start making physical activity part of your life, making it a priority and including it in your daily or weekly routine. When is the best time for you? Can you combine being active with something you already do, such as walking to work or going straight to an exercise class on your way home?	

Start low and build up slowly: Aim for realistic and achievable goals. A brisk 15 minute walk can eventually build up to a jog, and you can gradually increase the speed and distance. Avoid perfectionist or over-ambitious targets that put you off getting started.	
Make it social: Exercising with friends helps with motivation and enjoyment. Who can you enlist to go for a walk, join you at the gym or in a dance class?	
Focus on what's important: Choose activities based on what's important, realistic and helpful, and not based on whether you feel motivated to do it, which can fluctuate widely, depending on your mood.	
Think about the benefits: Picture yourself looking fitter and healthier and having more energy. Accept compliments from others and give yourself some encouraging words to keep going.	
Setbacks are normal! Expect setbacks and don't let these throw you permanently off track. On a busy week or if you are tired or injured, cut down to a low baseline, but try not to stop completely. Start building up again gradually when you are ready.	

Next steps for healthy activity habits

- What changes to your patterns of physical activity would be helpful in your life?

- Would you benefit from increasing moderate or vigorous activity and strengthening activities, or reducing time spent being sedentary?

- How might you get started?

- Can you fit in a short activity to break up your busy day? Think about making micro-changes rather than getting overwhelmed by perfectionist goals or plans.

6.5 Healthy eating habits

Good nutrition is important for both body and mind. There are many different approaches to healthy eating, which suit people with different bodies and lifestyles, and it's important to focus on what's helpful and realistic for you personally.

Finding healthy eating habits that work in your life will help you keep a healthy weight and provide energy to enjoy your daily activities. Making healthy eating choices can boost your self-esteem as you feel pride in choosing to take care of yourself, as well as reducing future health risks and modelling positive choices for others.

Eating and emotional wellbeing

Preparing food and eating together can be a time to appreciate and enjoy the moment and connect with friends and family. Try to use this as an opportunity to make healthy choices and seek out people who will support you in your healthy eating goals.

If you are feeling low or anxious, you may notice changes in your appetite or enjoyment of food. Some people turn to food as a comfort for emotional distress, which can lead to cravings for sugary or high fat junk foods. These may be enjoyable in the short term but have unhealthy consequences if they become a regular or frequent habit.

Eating disorders

It's important to recognise if you are struggling with an eating disorder, which can affect your physical health and emotional wellbeing. If eating makes you feel anxious, guilty or upset, or you are restricting your food intake or changing your eating patterns because of emotional distress, it is important to address this as there are effective treatments available. We recommend contacting your GP or seeking another form of support.

Motivate yourself with compassion

Thinking about changing your diet may sometimes trigger a barrage of self-critical or judgemental thoughts and strong emotions such as guilt and shame. This may contribute to unhealthy lifestyle choices as we may then turn to comfort eating as a way of numbing ourselves against emotional distress.

Rather than viewing healthy eating as restriction or a chore, each time you make a healthy choice, see it as a positive action, which represents giving yourself a gift of self-care. You are worth it! It can also be helpful to use **Open and Observe** skills as we pause, breathe, take a step back; recognising and acknowledging but not buying into any negative self-talk.

Helpful and unhelpful eating habits

Use the following table to reflect on the eating habits that are helpful and work well for you, and any unhelpful or unhealthy habits that you might wish to cut down or change:

Helpful and healthy eating habits	Unhelpful or unhealthy eating habits

PAUSE AND REFLECT: Why is healthy eating important to you?

Here are a few ideas to improve your healthy eating habits. Are any of these helpful or relevant?

Healthy eating habit	What's the first step towards this habit? What could you change or do differently?
Create a healthy routine: This might involve planning regular meals, having breakfast, intermittent fasting, or making choices about the type of food you wish to eat. Finding a healthy routine that is realistic and workable can help improve your mood and energy levels throughout the day.	
Overcome obstacles to healthy choices: For busy clinicians it can be a challenge to find time and access to healthy food choices. It may help to plan ahead and bring a healthy lunch to work. Cooking and freezing food in advance means that you are not coming home, tired and stressed, needing to cook from scratch at the end of the day when you lack energy.	

Eat for social connection or to take a pause: Avoid eating at your desk or 'on the go', when it's easy to make unhealthy choices and to not appreciate what you are eating. Make eating a time to pause or to connect with others. How could you make healthy choices at this time?	
Keep hydrated: Ensure you are drinking plenty of fluids through the day. Water helps hydrate you and may help to balance your appetite and food intake.	
Fill your cupboards with healthy food: This makes it easier to resist when you are tired or hungry. If you are tempted by the biscuit jar at work, try bringing in your own snacks or ask the practice manager to add something healthy alongside. Keep unhealthy snacks as an occasional treat rather than a regular habit.	

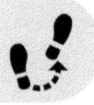

TAKE ACTION: Next steps for healthy eating habits

What small steps can you take towards creating healthy eating habits? This might involve anything from bringing healthy snacks or a packed lunch to work, improving your daily hydration patterns, to committing to eating a meal with your family each week.

- What will you try? Make a note of your thoughts here:

6.6 Healthy sleep habits

We all need good sleep, which is essential for rest and recuperation and for emotional and physical wellbeing. Lack of sleep and poor quality sleep can have many damaging effects, including weight gain, low mood and depression, poor performance and concentration, reduced creativity, and lower immunity to illness.

Stress, worry and low mood can affect sleep, as can stimulants such as caffeine, alcohol and drugs. Alcohol and certain drugs can become a 'false friend' – making you relaxed and sleepy at bedtime, but you then wake early or have disturbed sleep that is less refreshing.

For adults, the recommended amount of sleep is 7–8 hours, but this varies widely between individuals. The duration and quality of sleep can be affected by many factors, and there are many things you can do to improve your sleep.

Factors affecting sleep:

- Stressful life events
- Levels of daytime activity
- Circadian rhythm changes and shift-work patterns
- Physical symptoms such as pain at night
- Being kept awake by noise or light
- Carer duties overnight
- Sleep apnoea and snoring

How is your sleep?

The occasional poor night of sleep is completely normal. But, if you've been sleeping badly for a few weeks or longer, this may be a good time to look at what is triggering the disturbance and to make a change. The first step is to keep a track of your sleep amount and quality over one or two weeks:

Day/date	M	Tu	W	Th	F	Sa	Su
What time did you go to sleep?							
What time did you wake up?							
Rate the quality of your sleep: How rested or energetic did you feel afterwards? 1 - 2 - 3 - 4 - 5 - 6 - 7 - 8 - 9 - 10 ☹ 😊							
Notes: things that might have affected your sleep (helpful or unhelpful) or any disturbance to your routine							

Technology and sleep

Are your technology habits interfering with your sleep? Watching the news, checking emails or using social media late at night can make you feel agitated and alert, and interfere with sleep. Smartphones, tablets, computers and television screens also emit short-wavelength blue light, which may affect circadian rhythms and make you more alert at night.

Some tips for healthy screen use include:

- Cutting down late-night use of electronic devices, especially those which are held close to your face, such as phones and tablets
- Dimming the screen or using a night mode with warmer tones in the evening
- Listening to a relaxing audiobook rather than watching a screen at bedtime
- Charging your phone in another room or turning it off overnight, so that incoming messages and notifications don't affect your sleep.

Tips for improving sleep

Here are a few of our tips and strategies for improving your sleep patterns:

I have trouble getting to sleep	**Set a regular sleep pattern:** stick to similar times for going to bed and waking up each day and avoid sleeping in too long after a poor night's sleep or a late night. **Create a 'wind-down' routine:** plan a relaxing activity to prepare your body and mind for sleep, such as reading, listening to an audiobook, having a bath or doing yoga. **Make a 'sleep haven':** ensure your bedroom is dark, quiet and not too cluttered, that your bed is comfortable, and the room is a good temperature for sleeping. **Cut out daytime naps:** the odd nap after a late night is fine, but don't let this become a regular habit. If you really need to nap, make it short (15 minutes or less), and before 3 pm. **Reduce caffeine, nicotine, alcohol** or other stimulants, especially within 6 hours of bedtime. Avoid heavy meals late at night. **Cover the clock:** checking the time can lead to worry and impatience. Set the alarm and then wait until morning.
I have trouble staying asleep, or I wake early	**Sleep when you feel tired:** only try to sleep when you feel sleepy, rather than spending hours lying awake in bed. **Get up and try again later:** get up if you are still awake after around 20 minutes, and do something calming or boring, like sitting in a dimly lit room. Write down any thoughts that are troubling you and tell yourself you will revisit these in the morning. Return to bed when you feel sleepy and try to sleep again. Repeat the process if you still can't sleep. **Only use your bed for sleep, rest or sex:** have a separate desk or work area, and keep phones and computers out of the bedroom, if possible.
I have trouble waking up, or I wake up exhausted	**Avoid long lie-ins:** too much rest can make you more tired, particularly if you have low mood. **Regular daytime physical activity** keeps your body healthy and often helps more with fatigue than focusing on sleep. **Stick to your usual routine:** get up even if you are tired. Try taking a refreshing shower or doing a gentle yoga practice to liven you up.
I worry, have negative thoughts, dreams or memories that keep me awake or wake me up	**Low mood, trauma or anxiety can affect sleep:** look at the chapters in this book for some helpful ideas and share your concerns with a colleague or trusted friend. If necessary, seek professional help. **Write down problems or worries** in a journal or notebook. Do this well before bedtime and plan how you could cope with any difficulties. Use 'Thinking Time' if you are kept awake by an active mind (see *Chapter 9* on anxiety). **Don't try too hard:** you can't force yourself to sleep! Worrying about sleep will make you more anxious and keep you awake longer. Getting up for a short while might help. Remember, even a small amount of sleep is valuable. **You can cope better than you think:** a night without sleep is not a disaster. Think about ways of coping, taking care of yourself, and reducing demands the next day.

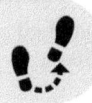

TAKE ACTION: Next steps for healthy sleep...

- What are your next steps to create healthy sleep habits?
- What small actions might help improve your sleep routine? This could be anything from increasing your daytime physical activity to planning a calming bedtime routine, where you put your phone out of sight and relax in a warm bath.

What will you try? Make a note of your thoughts here:

6.7 Other unhealthy habits

Substance and alcohol misuse can both cause physical and emotional damage and if you are affected, it's important to recognise the problem and seek help. You can find a list of helpful websites and organisations in the *Support for health professionals* section at the end of this book.

Technology habits

Living in a digital age brings many advantages but it can also be hard to keep track of or control how much time you are spending online. Overuse of technology can affect your productivity and memory, dampen creative thinking, increase stress and affect sleep.

Since the pandemic, patterns of remote working and home-schooling have increased screen use, as we use computers and phones to carry out remote consultations, check emails, messages, do online learning and interact with social media. While this can bring many benefits, it also increases the challenges of balancing time spent in front of a screen.

Technology use can start to become a problem if it's getting in the way of other important life activities. For example, smartphone use frequently involves short bursts of less than 30 seconds of activity, which may interfere with your focus on other tasks and distract you during face-to-face interactions. Screen time also keeps us sedentary, and reading negative news stories, or constantly comparing ourselves with others on social media, can lower our mood and self-esteem.

The aim is to balance your use of technology with other important parts of life, following your **Guide** as you make Wise choices about how to use your time. Using a screen time tracker can help you record how much time you are spending on a computer or phone, so you can decide if your patterns of screen use are slipping into unhealthy habits.

Next steps for healthy technology habits

How much time do you spend using technology or online? This might include:

- Working online, including emails, admin tasks and remote consultations
- Different platforms of social media
- Playing computer games
- Communicating via text messages or WhatsApp
- Facetime or video calls with friends or family.

PAUSE AND REFLECT: Balancing your technology habits

- What do you notice?
- Do you have the balance about right? Are your technology habits supporting wellbeing or do they get in the way of other life priorities?
- Do you use technology to avoid difficult feelings?
- Do you need to make any changes in your technology habits? What might be the first step?

Pressure and 'hurry habits'

Health professionals are usually extremely busy and we use our time to maximum effect at work. This can mean that the 'Drive' system we looked at in *Chapter 5* becomes overactive as you make a habit of filling every moment in your day. This might involve being over-ambitious with your capacity to do things outside of work as well. This is particularly true of people with perfectionist traits or who feel the urge to complete tasks or go above and beyond the call of duty. We feel pressured with time, constantly doing things at speed and with few pauses, and with reduced opportunity for enjoyment, relaxation and healthy choices.

Effective time management means allowing *enough* time, creating pauses in the day to allow you to recharge and nourish, whilst also allowing for unplanned and unexpected events. Things often take much longer than anticipated, and giving yourself unrealistic deadlines or planning in too many activities adds to stress and can increase the likelihood of things going wrong.

Here are some of our tips for managing time effectively:

Time management habits	What's the first step towards this habit? What could you change or do differently?
Slow down deliberately: remember to pause occasionally, take a breath and be mindful, allowing yourself time to gather your thoughts and re-energise.	
Make a plan and prioritise: make a realistic to-do list and record this using a diary, planner or calendar. Don't expect to achieve more than the 3 most important priorities on your list – anything else is a bonus!	
Leave space for the unexpected: ensure your schedule takes account of extra pressures or priorities such as traffic and the demands of others, as well as opportunities for spontaneous enjoyable activities like chatting with a friend.	
Manage your boundaries: it's sometimes essential to say 'no' to the demands of others and 'yes' to yourself when you need time alone or time for healthy habits. Delegating tasks involves sharing responsibility with colleagues, family and friends, and may help create some time for your personal needs.	

6.8 Caring for physical health

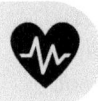

Looking after physical health is another way to care for your wellbeing. You may be living with a long-term condition or chronic physical health disorder, or simply looking for ways to stay healthy and reduce your risk of future health problems.

Living with a long-term condition can increase the risk of mental health difficulties such as low mood and anxiety. And if we become depressed or anxious, this also makes it harder to stick to the important self-care regimens that are necessary for effective management of our physical health. So, it's important to focus on our emotional wellbeing alongside managing physical health.

Boom–bust activity patterns

Slipping into a 'boom–bust' pattern of activity can undermine wellbeing, lead to physical deconditioning and worsen symptoms such as pain and fatigue.

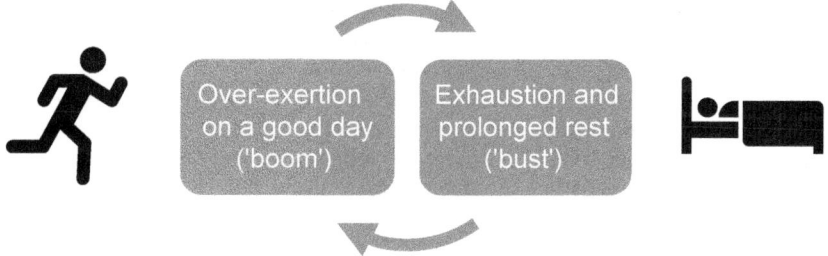

Whether you have a health problem or not, avoiding boom and bust is important for maintaining all healthy life habits. There are a few key principles:

- Make changes in activity gradual and realistic.

- Plan a baseline of minimum activity, such as ensuring that you move every 20–30 minutes, that you can manage even on a bad day, and try to stick to this.

- If you are busy or under pressure, try cutting back your expectations, or halving your usual exercise, rather than stopping completely.

- Have a plan for coping, building up gradually again after a setback such as illness or injury.

PAUSE AND REFLECT: Tips for managing a physical health condition

Here are some of our tips for maintaining your physical and emotional wellbeing:

Managing physical health habits	What's the first step towards this? What could you change or do differently?
Do what matters most: rather than trying to do everything, prioritise values such as self-care, acceptance and important relationships, which move you towards making your health a priority.	
Focus on quality of life: don't make healthy living a chore. To lift your mood as well as improve physical health, ensure that you include a range of activities that are meaningful and enjoyable.	

Check in with your emotions: living with health problems can lower your mood, and cause frustration and irritability. Physical activity may provide a release. Taking time to notice and acknowledge our emotions and sharing them with trusted people may also help.	
Be compassionate: remember how your patients at work appreciate and respond to empathy and support. How can you be compassionate or show yourself care?	
Acceptance: this is not about giving up or giving in. It's about acknowledging what you have control over. You may not be able to change an underlying health problem, but it is in your power to change your reactions. You can choose helpful and positive actions that are likely to maximise your wellbeing and quality of life.	
Patience and perseverance: it may take longer than you would like to make healthy changes and stick to them. You may also need to pause and be patient during a flare-up or relapse, as you adjust to changing circumstances whilst continuing to follow your **Guide** as you reset your routine.	

6.9 Overcoming unhelpful life habits

Maybe you have reached this section and are thinking: "Actually, I think I'm OK. I have a fairly good balance, and I think I'm doing fine!" Or maybe you are caught up a vicious cycle, with some unhealthy life habits getting out of balance, in which case you might find it helpful to pause and reflect further.

Thoughts, feelings and behaviours

Certain thoughts, feelings, behaviours, people and places can create obstacles to us in seeing through our intentions, setting goals and creating healthy life habits. They can create unhelpful patterns and vicious cycles which keep us stuck and unable to take steps. There are also things that help or enable us to change. Use the following table to list any thoughts and feelings, behaviours or situations that make it harder to stick to healthy life habits. We will look at some ways to tackle these using **GROWTH** skills in the next section:

What gets in the way of making a change?	What are your own examples?	What can you change? What might help with this?
Difficult thoughts and feelings e.g. I feel too tired; I can't do it well enough; I'm too stressed; it's impossible		
Situations or places e.g. after a long day at work; when I'm busy with family life; when other people are having a glass of wine or eating unhealthy food; bad weather		
Behaviours and habits e.g. turning the alarm off at the weekend; shopping when I'm hungry; eating late at night; rushing		

6.10 GROWTH skills for healthy life habits

In this section we will summarise the key **GROWTH** skills to help you create healthy life habits and routines.

Use your Guide

The first step is to turn to your inner **Guide** to find motivation and decide what's important. Which healthy life habit do you wish to focus on? What are the reasons for this? What are the benefits and why does it matter to you?

If negative thoughts get in the way, try to remind yourself of the reasons for making a change, and your longer-term goals. Think about how you would like to see yourself, both now and in the future.

Ready for action

Don't wait to feel motivated before you get started with **Healthy Life Habits**. We sometimes don't feel like doing things but may feel great afterwards. You might experience a barrage of negative thoughts such as:

I can't be bothered! I'm too tired! I hate exercise!

This is impossible, I'll never manage it, so there's no point trying…

Instead of allowing these thoughts to pull you back into an old unhealthy habit, try choosing to take one small healthy action, even if the negative thoughts are there. Start by planning one realistic goal. What's the first small step? What would make it easier to get started? For example, committing to meet a friend to do a workout in the park.

Choose a goal that will be likely to keep you feeling positive and enthusiastic. It's helpful to plan ahead and make the goal specific and concrete by making a note in your calendar, diary or phone. What's your plan B if things have to adjust slightly?

Open and Observe

Stay **Open and Observe** and acknowledge any negative thoughts, or distressing or painful feelings, that may be creating an obstacle to your healthy life plan. Perhaps your inner critic tends to step in when you contemplate making a change, such as:

> I'm so unfit, I'll look ridiculous. I haven't played sport for years – I'm useless at it!

> I'm far too busy with work and my family life!

Can you create a short pause to step back and observe your inner experiences, enabling you to 'surf' the urge pulling you back towards unhealthy choices? It's not necessary to argue, criticise or blame yourself for finding this hard. Instead, try engaging with your five senses, or using 'notice the NOW' to create some stability and choice.

Try also to notice any people or places that make it harder to change, and think about practical ways to support yourself to make more healthy choices.

Wise Mind

Let your **Wise Mind** take a lead in what's most helpful for you. Listen to your inner coach, making Wise choices that follow your inner **Guide**. Planning your time and creating a structure can help reduce stress, and continuing actions regularly will help to form a healthy habit.

If you are struggling to find the time to fit in activities such as physical exercise, remind yourself that prioritising time for you is essential. It's important to find a balance between work and self-care, and without it you will be less effective. A 5 or 10 minute burst of activity can improve your focus and attention and help get more done.

Thrive and Balance

Keeping your three emotion systems balanced involves using the drive system to motivate yourself to make important health changes, whilst giving enough time to the calm and connect system for rest and recuperation. It's also important to manage the threat system so you are not too stressed, anxious or overwhelmed to keep up these important activities. This may mean keeping your drive system in check by being realistic about how much you can reasonably expect yourself to achieve each day.

Use self-compassion to help you cope with any difficult feelings that arise when you are making a change. Perhaps there is discomfort from perfectionist ideas about what you 'should' be able to achieve, or guilt as you pull back from over-drive and over-work and place much-needed focus on your own needs. Try to be kind to yourself and set realistic and fair goals that are 'good enough'. Remember common humanity – we are all struggling with keeping a balance, and it's impossible to do everything. We can only do the best we can and be kind to ourselves in the process.

Can you plan some calm and soothing activities and create some 'pauses' in your day to help you get a little more balance and perspective?

Healthy Life Habits

Building a routine by structuring activities and planning your time can help to make healthy choices a part of your life, reducing stress and making it easier to fit things into a busy schedule. It's also important to prioritise. Choose activities based on what's important and meaningful and follow your inner **Guide** as you put yourself and your wellbeing at the top of the list – create personal *non-negotiables*.

What are your non-negotiables? These are activities that you always make time for, no matter what else is happening. They include activities like showering, going to work, eating, childcare duties and sleeping.

You can choose to make any activity one of your personal non-negotiables. This can include healthy life habits and prioritising your health and wellbeing. You may decide to adjust how much time you spend on them each day, but they will remain part of your regular routine.

After planning your non-negotiables, you can decide what else you want to achieve each day. Ask yourself: how *important* and *urgent* is each activity? Does it have to be done today? Try to include no more than three priority items on your to-do list that are urgent for each day, along with your non-negotiables.

Non-negotiable activities	Priority activities (no more than 3 per day)	Other activities (not urgent for today)

It is also important to be realistic about how long things take and allow for unexpected events or problems. So, it helps not to cram too much onto your to-do list. It may also help to create an 'If… then…' plan to overcome likely problems or obstacles for healthy habits:

- *If it's not raining, then I will cycle to work. If it's raining, then I will do 10 minutes on my exercise bike in the garage when I get home.*

- *If I'm working a long day, then I will break it up with some short walks to re-energise.*

- *If I'm feeling hungry at work, then I will eat a healthy snack and have a glass of water.*

- *If I'm tempted to check my emails or Twitter late at night, then I will put on an audiobook instead.*

Moving from consciously planning healthy choices to creating a Healthy habit is simple: REPEAT + REPEAT + REPEAT! Make this a non-negotiable part of your routine.

Penny reflects: *"My inner Guide is pointing towards taking better care of myself and being a role model for my daughters. I really want them to develop a healthy relationship with food and with being active. I also want to look after my physical health. My mum has diabetes with complications, and I want to take action before I reach the same point.*

When I think about trying to lose weight it's easy to feel hopeless. I get a lot of negative thoughts predicting that I will 'fail' at yet another diet, and I start to feel despondent and ashamed of my inability to change. I then have an urge to give up and eat a whole packet of biscuits, or else I get lost on Twitter as a way to distract myself.

I tried using an Open and Observe practice to notice and name how I was feeling, and I recognised some strong emotions and tried to accept and acknowledge these. After a pause, I was also able to notice that my technology habits are making me more sedentary as well as making me stressed and disconnected from my family.

I feel a bit overwhelmed, there seem to be so many changes I need to make. But I like the idea of asking my Wise self to make decisions, and to be more compassionate. I've always made changes from a negative perspective, but now I'm planning to change because I care about myself and my wellbeing.

I'm going to focus on making a few small realistic changes. I will focus on the benefits of looking after my health and try to make some wise choices on how I use my time. I am also going to make it a habit to plan our family activities for the week together on a Sunday evening and make sure I include some time for myself in the week.

I'm thinking of investing in a standing desk – I've always wanted one! I'm also planning to try and involve my daughters in cooking healthily as a family – giving us time to connect and making it more fun for everyone.

My friend has asked me to train with her on a Couch to 5k jogging plan. I think that sounds a bit hard for me – but I will meet her in the park, and we can do a walking warm-up together which would be nice. Maybe I can build my confidence to do more in time!"

Chapter summary: Healthy Life Habits

- **GROWTH** steps can help create realistic **Healthy Life Habits** which balance a healthy lifestyle with work, relationships and family commitments.
    - ○ Follow your inner **Guide** to find motivation and decide what's important
    - ○ Get **Ready for action** by planning small actions that prioritise your wellbeing
    - ○ Observing and accepting negative thoughts and painful feelings enables greater choice as you learn to surf unhealthy behavioural urges
    - ○ Let your **Wise Mind** take a lead in what's most helpful for you personally
    - ○ **Thrive** as you approach healthy living with self-compassion rather than self-criticism or blame
    - ○ Prioritise and repeat healthy actions so they become part of your routine.

Final thoughts

What are the most important messages for you from this chapter?

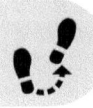

Take an action step

What are your next steps? What actions will you take as a result of reading this chapter?

What concrete steps can you take towards building **Healthy Life Habits** that are meaningful in your life?

07 Personality traits and traps

- Do you take on tasks and responsibilities even when you don't have capacity, time or energy, at the expense of your own rest, leisure and sleep?

- Do you put yourself under extreme pressure to meet high standards and then become exhausted or self-critical if things don't go completely to plan?

- Do you compare yourself negatively to colleagues, or are you constantly waiting to be found out as an imposter who doesn't deserve admiration or praise?

- Let's look at some common personality traits and how we can work to our strengths whilst avoiding some of their potential traps...

7.1 Personality traits: strengths and vulnerabilities

Personality traits are patterns of thoughts, feelings and behaviour, which influence our values, attitudes, motivations and coping strategies at work and in our personal lives. These characteristics are influenced by multiple factors, including genetics, family environment and life experiences, and exert a powerful influence on the work-related wellbeing of health professionals (Blackwelder *et al.*, 2016).

Primary care clinicians are typically compassionate, caring, reliable people who take great pride in their work. Our roles involve balancing clinical skills, knowledge and experience, with the ability to analyse, draw conclusions, make decisions, show empathy and communicate effectively. Yet the very traits that create excellent clinicians, such as conscientiousness, attention to detail, and high personal standards, may also bring challenges if they become rigid or extreme. These traits can become personality 'traps' which pull us into unhealthy patterns of behaviour, trigger high levels of emotional arousal, and create an increased vulnerability to stress and burnout.

Working to our strengths involves acknowledging and accepting our own personality traits, without allowing them to become extreme, rigid or unhelpful. This can help us to live in line with our values, reach our potential at work and in our home life, and find ways to thrive in the face of stress and challenge.

In this chapter we look at:

- Understanding common personality 'traps' such as perfectionism, obsessional focus, imposter syndrome and being a 'chronic hero'.

- Exploring how these traits may influence how we work and relate to others.

- Using the **GROWTH** skills that we discussed in the earlier chapters to maximise our strengths, support areas of vulnerability, and improve our quality of life and wellbeing.

Let's look at some examples of how personality traits might affect members of the primary care team. Can you recognise which of our professionals might fall into the traps of perfectionism, being a chronic hero, or imposter syndrome?

Siobhan, Nurse Manager: *"I like to do things well and don't feel satisfied until I am certain that everything is exactly right."*

Neelam, Practice Nurse: *"I often feel anxious at work, and worry that my colleagues are doing a better job than I am. I'm sure one day I'll get found out or make a major mistake and everyone will realise that I'm not really fit for the job..."*

Matthew, Salaried GP: *"I'm so used to saying 'yes' that I hardly even think about it. I feel guilty if I take time off, so I end up over-working and never seem to find time to take care of myself."*

7.2 Unhealthy perfectionism

What is perfectionism?

Being perfectionist involves relentlessly pursuing personally demanding standards, and basing your self-worth on achieving them, which negatively affects wellbeing. People sometimes say, 'I can't possibly be a perfectionist... I'm so untidy!'. Yet there are many types of perfectionism with expectations about achievement in different domains, including being liked by others or not making mistakes.

Perfectionism or high standards?

It's important for health professionals to have high standards, including attention to detail and a healthy desire to get things right. These valuable traits contribute to a sense of accomplishment and self-esteem, and are associated with values such as achievement, pursuing excellence and developing skills and expertise, and beliefs such as:

- It's good to go home knowing I've completed all my work

- I like to do things well

- I get satisfaction from knowing I tried my hardest

- It's better to be prepared for unexpected problems.

Maintaining healthy high standards involves being able to relax, adapt or flex them when needed. This allows us to be realistic about our expectations and maintain a balance between meeting the demands of complex situations and our own needs. In contrast, perfectionism can involve unreasonable standards which are impossible to consistently achieve in the real world, so we are setting ourselves up to fail. Trying to live up to these rigid rules, demands or expectations has a negative impact on our lives and self-esteem.

Siobhan, Nurse Manager: Siobhan was promoted last year and is responsible for managing a team of nurse practitioners, practice nurses and healthcare assistants in a large GP practice. She is conscientious and cares deeply about her professional life. She works long hours and does not rest until she is sure that the team has met or exceeded their targets. She can become frustrated and irritable with colleagues when others don't match her high standards.

"I like to do things well and I don't feel satisfied until I am certain that everything is running smoothly in the team. I sometimes end up doing tasks myself and working long days because colleagues haven't done things in exactly the right way. Sometimes I don't get home until it's time to go to bed and then I'm too frustrated to sleep!"

The costs of perfectionism

The relentless pursuit of demanding standards in perfectionism can contribute to burnout, insomnia, anxiety and depression. We may over-work, plan and organise excessively, and struggle to delegate tasks, as we want them to be absolutely 'right'.

The paradox of perfectionism is that extreme high standards can actually get in the way of achieving goals. When we place ourselves under enormous pressure, the stress, anxiety and fear of failure make it harder to perform at a high standard. We start to feel overwhelmed, procrastinate, have difficulty making decisions, work more slowly, and avoid or give up in the face of challenges.

Perfectionism and self-esteem

Perfectionists tend to judge their self-worth based on their ability to achieve. So, if things go wrong, even if for reasons outside their control, perfectionists may resort to self-blame or start to view themselves as worthless or as a failure, with feelings of sadness, shame and despair.

When perfectionist standards are met, there may be a short-lived sense of relief, but there is often a tendency to re-evaluate the original standard as 'not high enough' so self-criticism returns, with nothing ever quite feeling good enough.

Siobhan reflects on the benefits and challenges of her high standards:

"I was praised at my recent appraisal for my committed attitude and excellent work, and I'm sure that's why I was offered this role, even though I'm younger than some of the other nurses in the team. I get a lot of satisfaction from completing my work and knowing I have given it my best.

But having high standards can be difficult. Like most people, I had never faced a situation like working through the pandemic, and I wanted to show I could rise to the challenge. But some of my team had other priorities such as families or stresses at home and were less focused on work. I was new to managing a team, and I found it hard when I met resistance or others didn't meet my expectations. I started sacrificing my own time until I was sure everything was done, but the increasing workload is now making this much harder to achieve. I know this is starting to affect me."

Spotting unhealthy perfectionism

PAUSE AND REFLECT: Noticing perfectionism

Take a look at some of the following perfectionist beliefs and traits. Add comments next to any that you can relate to. What's the impact of holding this belief – what do you typically do as a result? Are there any costs to holding this belief, at work, home or in other areas of your life?

Perfectionist beliefs and traits	What do you typically do as a result?	Are there any costs to you at work or in your wider life?
Nothing good comes from making mistakes. I must do things right first time.	EXAMPLE: I put off starting tasks until I think I can do it correctly	My to-do list gets longer and I feel stressed
I have to go over my work many times until it seems good enough.		

If I can't do something perfectly, there's no point in trying.		
I rarely give myself credit when I do well because I could always do more. No achievement ever feels enough.		
Sometimes I'm so concerned about getting one task done perfectly that I don't have time to complete the rest of my work.		
People tend to think my expectations of them are too high or too rigid.		
I put off starting things because I want things to be perfect or I'm worried about failing.		
I don't trust others to do a good job, so I prefer not to delegate and end up doing things myself.		
I like to go to bed leaving no tasks undone. Sometimes I can't sleep for worrying whether I've made mistakes or not completed everything.		

Siobhan notices that she holds several perfectionist beliefs which have triggered some unhelpful behaviour patterns:

"Because I don't trust anyone else to do a good job, I often end up doing it all myself, so I have very little free time to relax at home. I used to have a good

social life and a supportive girlfriend, but now I have no time for relationships or leisure.

My sleep is a problem and I'm often tired, which makes it harder to concentrate during the day. I go to bed late because I try to complete all my housework before bed, and then I lie awake worrying about anything I haven't done well enough, especially at work.

I also know that I can be hard on my colleagues. I'd really like to improve my relationships with other members of my team."

Obsessional focus

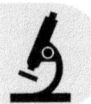

Some people with perfectionism may also recognise the trap of 'obsessional focus'. Like all the personality traits, it brings many positive qualities, but can cause challenges if it becomes an extreme or rigid behaviour pattern.

People with obsessional focus traits are often high achievers who appear confident and organised, with meticulous standards that enable them to perform their role to an extremely high standard. They are hard-working, reliable, productive and conscientious. But the downsides of this trait include tending to prioritise work over relationships, and we may get so caught up in rules and schedules that we lose the purpose of what we're doing or become highly distressed when things don't go as planned.

There can also be challenges in relationships. People with obsessional focus may struggle to empathise or see other people's perspectives and perceive their own view as the only 'right' way to see a situation. This can be exhausting and frustrating for colleagues and partners.

Obsessional focus is particularly challenging if it comes hand in hand with anxiety and difficulty tolerating uncertainty. High levels of focus and attention can slip into constant rumination and excessive preoccupation, making it harder to engage with other valued life areas such as family, relationships or leisure.

Recognising obsessional focus

PAUSE AND REFLECT: Traits of obsessional focus

Take a look at the following questions and consider whether you recognise any traits of obsessional focus:

Obsessional focus beliefs and traits	What do you typically do as a result?	Are there any costs to you at work or in your wider life?
I prioritise conscientiousness and dedication to work at the expense of other aspects of daily life	Example: I often find myself working until late at night	I miss out on time with my partner and family
I have a strong interest in order, details, lists and organisation		
I prefer to follow rules exactly as they are written		
I often consider my own perspective as being the best or only way to approach a problem or situation		
I find it difficult to change my attitude or compromise		
I find it hard to see the world from other people's perspectives		
I have high expectations of others and can be critical if these are not met		
I find it difficult to give up control or to delegate tasks		
I find it hard to make decisions because I want them to be 'right'		
I often get stuck or preoccupied with thoughts about work, or specific tasks or problems		

Some of the traits of obsessional focus may also arise in people with traits of autism, and if you strongly recognise these, it may also be helpful to explore this possibility in more detail.

GROWTH skills for perfectionism and obsessional focus

Use your inner Guide

It's great to have high standards, but not for them to be so extreme that they reduce your wellbeing or enjoyment of life. Think about your inner **Guide** and who you want to be as a person. Can you hold any values that relate to high standards and achievement more lightly and balance these with other important values such as relationships, self-care and relaxation?

PAUSE AND REFLECT: What are your values?

Think about your wider values, your personal needs, and notice which direction your inner **Guide** is pointing. Now ask yourself:

- What's most important to you? What do you value in life?
- Is the pursuit of unrelenting standards getting in the way of living fully according to your values?
- Are you prioritising certain values to the exclusion of others?

Ready for Action

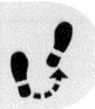

Perfectionists are great at taking action but often get overburdened with excessive tasks and expectations and may try to fit too much in. Can you reduce a goal to make it more manageable and achievable?

If we measure our success and self-worth purely by achievements and results, we may become stressed and overwhelmed by our expectations. Instead, you can focus on the process rather than the outcome. Setting goals that involve participating in activities rather than being 'good' at them can ease the pressure and may even help you reach a higher standard in the long term. For example, you might plan to engage in daily physical activity without setting pressurised goals for how far or fast you 'should' run or swim.

Try doing things for fun or because you've always wanted to try them, rather than because you're good at them, or are striving for achievement or praise. Some things are worth trying, even if the outcome is imperfect.

It can also be helpful to create reasonable boundaries around certain activities. Just because you have set an expectation to complete every task by the end of the working day, does not mean you have to rigidly follow this. Can you experiment with flexing or changing your rules and expectations? Could you try adapting a rigid routine, whilst finding ways to self-care and tolerate any distress or discomfort that may accompany the change?

Try something new for fun, without having a specific outcome or target – just to see how it feels. Make a plan for when you will do this, who with, and for how long.

Open and Observe

Observe when a perfectionist belief is being activated and take a moment to notice and name your thoughts, feelings, body sensations and urges to take action. Try using a brief mindfulness exercise from *Chapter 3* to make space for the belief, without acting on it immediately.

Can you practise softening or relaxing one of your perfectionist rules, just a little, allowing yourself more space to be human and fallible? Can you experiment with doing something to an 'OK', 'good enough' or 'reasonable' standard? Try aiming for silver or bronze rather than a gold medal? What would 70% effort and achievement look like? Could this be enough – at least sometimes?

Siobhan's Example:

The perfectionist beliefs I notice are: I must keep exactly to time on all appointments, and I insist that others in the team do the same.

I am going to allow myself some space and relax this belief: I will make this a 'preference' rather than being too exact and allow myself a few minutes leeway. When I tried this, I found I felt less stressed, was able to focus more clearly and that things worked out without major delays.

PAUSE AND REFLECT: Complete the following:

The perfectionist beliefs I notice are:

I am going to allow myself some space and relax this belief by:

Use Wise Mind

Our perfectionist part brings many skills and positive attributes, but it's not necessary to allow it to dominate or control you entirely. Instead, invite your wise mind or inner coach to step up and act as a leader, who acknowledges the contributions of the perfectionist traits, but who takes a kinder and more realistic perspective when planning goals and expectations.

Would you benefit from developing a growth mindset, which recognises that we continually learn and develop with time, effort and practice? Here, success is less about proving that you're smart or talented and more about stretching yourself to learn something new. This makes it easier to take on challenges, as we start to see failure as merely a temporary setback and the starting point for developing new abilities and skills. We talk more about a growth mindset in *Chapter 12*.

Thrive and Balance and Healthy Life Habits

Perfectionism is often fuelled by self-criticism, and learning to relate to yourself with kindness can help to quieten our negative inner voice. We can use self-compassion to develop acceptance of our imperfections and flaws, allowing ourselves to let go of demanding or unrealistic expectations.

At times that you are struggling, try to imagine what an understanding or supportive friend might say. It can also be helpful to find ways to soothe distressing emotions, such as listening to music or going for a walk in the countryside. Take a look at the three circles model from *Section 5.6* for ideas on how to build your skills in self-compassion and have more balance between the threat, drive and soothe systems.

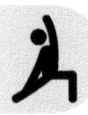

Finally, think about your patterns of living. What routines, structures or healthy life choices might support you in feeling happier, more balanced and content in your daily life? Can you plan to make even small changes that move you towards these often neglected values and needs?

Siobhan applies some GROWTH skills:

"I realised that I wasn't following my inner Guide, especially in values of caring for myself and others, which brought me into this profession in the first place. I felt bad about some of my angry outbursts – this isn't how I want to be as a colleague or a manager.

I took some time out at the weekend and went for a walk with my sister. Instead of pretending everything was fine, I shared with her how hard I've been finding things. She is always a good listener, and she helped me see how some of my perfectionist traits have got out of hand, and my life is out of balance.

I decided to try and create a more supportive and effective team at work, by involving my colleagues more and planning some team meetings. I might ask

> *the practice manager whether I could look for some leadership training. I also set limits on my working hours, making sure I don't stay late every day. I will try to get some enjoyment in my life by arranging a meal with friends at least once a week. I might even take a sculpture class – I've always wanted to try it and I've never done it before!"*

7.3 Imposter syndrome

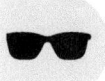

People with imposter syndrome, which is surprisingly common amongst high achievers, experience persistent self-doubt and fear of being exposed as a fraud. You may be outwardly successful, yet continue to doubt your ability and talent, attributing your achievements to error or luck, rather than personal qualities such as intelligence, skills or experience.

Personality traits associated with imposter syndrome can create a chronic sense of stress which affects job performance, job satisfaction and wellbeing, and increases the risk of stress and burnout.

Neelam, practice nurse: Neelam has been a practice nurse at a busy surgery for 5 years and recently qualified as a nurse prescriber. Patients often remark on her friendly, empathetic style, and will frequently ask to see her in preference to other clinicians. She is also well-liked and highly valued by her colleagues and the practice manager. However, Neelam often feels anxious at work despite having a supportive team and receiving positive feedback from both patients and colleagues.

"I just don't feel I deserve people's respect and praise. Instead, I often feel overwhelmed and question whether I know what I'm doing. This means I end up working really hard and longer hours. It's probably because I work so hard that I've been lucky, and they haven't seen through me. I keep thinking I'll make a significant or even fatal mistake one day and then people will realise that I'm a fraud and not fit for the job."

Negative self-beliefs and discounting achievements

People with imposter syndrome tend to hold beliefs about not being good enough, or not measuring up to the standards of others. When faced by challenging situations such as making a mistake, receiving a small criticism, being asked to do a presentation, taking an exam, or applying for a new role, an individual with imposter syndrome may experience a barrage of negative thoughts and fears. To compensate for their perceived 'flaws', the individual often develops perfectionist beliefs and rules.

Even when things go well, imposter beliefs can interfere with the ability to accept and enjoy achievements. We minimize our successes and use our hard work as evidence that whilst we 'got away with it' this time, we don't really deserve praise or recognition.

Neelam: *"I was convinced I would fail the assessment for my nurse prescriber qualification. I worked extremely hard, and I got a good mark, although I found it very stressful. Now I think it was a complete fluke which I only achieved through cramming and hard work. I will never be as competent as my colleagues and I'm dreading the personal development review that's due soon. I never ask questions in case people realise that I haven't really got what it takes. I'm sure they feel sorry for me and that's why they try to reassure me and say I'm doing OK."*

The impact of imposter syndrome

Imposter syndrome tends to become more obvious when we are facing an achievement-based task which feels outside our comfort zone, such as taking on a new role or responsibilities. We respond by avoiding these kinds of threatening or challenging situations. So, we don't go for a promotion or take on a leadership role and shy away from giving a presentation at work. This may reduce short-term anxiety, but also reinforces self-doubting beliefs, limits opportunities for development and reduces wellbeing.

You may also feel the need to 'prove yourself' by over-working. Perhaps you avoid asking for help or sharing your feelings, for fear of revealing your flaws to others. Or you may find yourself over-preparing, working gruelling hours, or putting excessive time or effort into projects, which interferes with other priorities in life.

EXERCISE: Do you struggle with feeling like an 'imposter'?

Can you recognise any of the following beliefs and traits that are commonly associated with imposter syndrome?

Beliefs and traits	What do you typically do as a result?	What are the costs at work or in your wider life?
I often think I'm a fraud and live in fear of being found out	Example: I'm constantly stressed and feel I have to perform things really well	I feel stressed and anxious a lot of the time and this is exhausting

Even when I do well, I don't think I really deserve it and put it down to luck rather than ability or talent		
I find it hard to accept praise or compliments and downplay my achievements		
I see my colleagues as more competent or intelligent than me		
I shy away from challenges and opportunities or sharing my ideas because of self-doubt		
If I show 'weakness' or ask others for help they may think less of me		
I need to use charm, or work extra hard, to make sure I'm not 'found out'		
I feel uncomfortable if I have to speak with experts such as consultants or professors		

GROWTH skills for imposter syndrome

Use your inner Guide

Instead of being over-focused on protecting your self-image and hiding possible flaws, can you turn to your inner **Guide** to identify any personal values that might be more important or meaningful? Focusing on values such as collaboration, connection, openness and teamwork can reduce feelings of separation and difference. This helps you to collaborate and work more closely with colleagues on shared goals and achievements.

Ready for Action

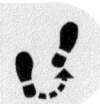

It's completely normal to sometimes doubt yourself, feel anxious and to have thoughts about being an imposter. But it's important not to allow these thoughts to control your behaviour. Instead, you can choose confident actions, where you behave 'as if' you believe in yourself and your abilities. What would you do if you felt (a little) more confident? What small steps would you take? Think of someone that you admire who demonstrates confident behaviour – what would they do? Can you try this, even if you are experiencing anxiety or self-doubt?

Open and Observe

Open up to others: we often keep imposter syndrome hidden, putting on a 'mask' of competency in front of others, so our imposter beliefs are never challenged. Try letting down your guard a little, perhaps by showing some vulnerability, asking for help, or admitting that you find something difficult. Can you find fun and laughter using light-hearted humour to reveal some of your imperfections?

It may help to confide in a trusted colleague or mentor, who may often have similar inner imposter beliefs. Knowing that others share your feelings can help to normalise your experiences and gain some perspective.

Observe imposter beliefs: notice and name when imposter beliefs and feelings pop up, saying to yourself: "I'm having thoughts about being a fraud. I'm feeling anxious about being found out by my colleagues". Observing rather than engaging with the thought can create some distance and perspective. Take a look at *Chapter 3* for a reminder of Observe skills to help you step back from unhelpful thoughts and strong emotions.

Wise Mind

Your **Wise Mind** can help you respond more positively to challenges and notice when your 'negative filter' is switched on. Next time imposter beliefs or feelings pop up, ask yourself: how would a supportive, caring friend or colleague view this situation? What would they advise you? Is this imposter belief helping you? If not, what would be a more helpful and balanced perspective?

To counter self-doubt, spend 5 minutes each day seeking evidence of your own competence and success. Use a daily 'skills journal' to make a note of even small achievements, noting down specific events that demonstrate your abilities. What skills or personal qualities can you recognise? Include any positive feedback that you have received from patients and colleagues, no matter how small this is. This is a cumulative process of building your observations using many examples of your skills and abilities.

Thrive and Balance and Healthy Life Habits

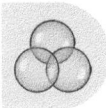

Try to keep your threat–drive systems in balance by bringing in care and compassion. Seek a sense of common humanity, which recognises that as health professionals, we all wish to do our best, but having flaws and imperfections is part of being human. Allowing others to share their knowledge and skills can help you to work more collaboratively, and balance the drive system, without getting stuck in over-drive to 'prove yourself', and overcoming procrastination if you feel stuck or overwhelmed.

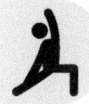

Also think about making healthy life choices and not neglecting the need for physical activity, social interaction and relaxation, without this becoming another demand. What small changes might move you towards this?

Neelam uses her GROWTH skills: *"This week it all got too much. I was struggling with the IT system because I was never shown how to use the computer and it kept crashing! I felt stressed and overwhelmed. I wasn't sure what to do, but I decided to pause between patients and try the NOW technique (see Section 3.2) that I had used once before. It only took a few minutes to get things back in check. When I was thinking more clearly, I noticed I was having the thought that I 'should' know how to use the computer better. I used* **Wise Mind** *and relaxed this rule, took a breath, and then decided to be brave and ask for help. I told Carol on reception the reason for my delayed appointments and asked her to warn patients. I felt embarrassed but I also asked if she had any advice. Her response was not what I expected. She said that many staff struggle and there is usually an induction to get to grips with the system. The admin staff had thought I was so high tech and were really impressed I'd been using it without training. We had a bit of a laugh and I felt very supported. Admitting I was struggling and asking for help has spurred me on to try this more often. I want to do this job well, and I really want to give myself the chance."*

7.4 The 'chronic hero': excessive responsibility and guilt

Most health professionals are compassionate and caring people who take great pride in their work. Yet many excellent, responsible, caring doctors also struggle with inappropriate, irrational guilt and an exaggerated sense of duty. This may create a 'chronic hero', who has an overwhelming desire to fix everything that goes wrong and who believes they are somehow responsible for things that are beyond their control.

A healthy level of guilt can be advantageous for clinicians working in 'helping professions', encouraging qualities such as respect, empathy, professionalism and dedication. However, too much guilt takes its toll, and we may start to place undue pressure on ourselves, become self-critical, and worry that we have never done as much as we 'should'.

Matthew is a salaried GP who has always loved his job and been very committed to his career. In the past, he felt motivated, energetic and enthusiastic, but lately he has been working extra hours due to staff shortages, feeling it was his duty to help out. Now he is struggling with fatigue and is finding it hard to balance work with other commitments. Matthew's elderly mother is unwell with dementia, but lives far away and his father is struggling to cope. As the only child, Matthew feels a great sense of responsibility for their wellbeing. He has given up many leisure activities such as swimming and Parkruns and feels guilty if he takes time to himself or goes to meet friends.

"I am so used to saying yes to extra duties that I don't even think about it – I just get on with it. My colleagues and patients need me to help. I feel guilty when I have a day off and most weekends I drive to visit my parents, so I never get a break. I know the advice about regular time for yourself, exercise and a healthy diet, but what if you have many responsibilities and little time? My approach is to grab some fast food when I leave work and push myself harder to get all my work done so I can visit my parents each week."

Getting stuck as a 'chronic hero'

Constant striving to be a hero in the workplace can lead to over-work, perfectionism and guilt over every problem that arises. The continual sense of pressure to help others can be exhausting and puts a strain on the hero's personal life.

'Chronic heroes' are often motivated by helping others, but their actions may not always be beneficial. Having 'chronic heroes' amongst leaders and managers may create an unhealthy culture of invulnerability in workplaces, which makes it harder for others to admit when they are struggling. Hero-type behaviour may also create dependency and disempowerment in patients and colleagues, undermining the other person's belief in their ability to cope. Heroes are also at greater risk of becoming drawn into manipulative relationships.

When facing mistakes or complaints, heroes often feel extreme guilt and shame for having 'failed' to save the day. Heroes may also be vulnerable to distress from moral injury in situations which violate our moral or ethical code. So, when we see health systems or services that are struggling or unable to provide effective care, we may internalise the blame, with powerful feelings of inner guilt and personal responsibility for being unable to do more.

Matthew – a 'chronic hero'

"I don't seem to be able to stop myself taking on extra duties, even though I'm not a partner and many of these issues are not my responsibility. When we were short-staffed, I offered to work an extra day, although I had been due to meet an old friend. I feel very guilty about many of my patients who weren't seen during the pandemic and feel responsible for making it up to them.

Now the pressure is starting to get to me, and I've made a few silly mistakes – missing some abnormal blood results. Luckily nothing serious so far but I'm worried it may get worse. And my health and relationships are suffering. I'm tired and irritable, and I've started to resent the demands of some 'worried well' patients. I compare them with my parents who are frail and struggling, and I feel angry and frustrated. A patient even complained to the receptionist about my abruptness the other day. This just isn't me...."

EXERCISE: Could you be a 'chronic hero'?

Consider the beliefs and actions of Matthew in the example above. Can you recognise any of the following beliefs that are commonly held by people with 'chronic hero' traits?

Beliefs and traits	What do you typically do as a result?	What are the costs to you at work or in your wider life?
I volunteer to take on responsibilities even if they are not mine	Example: I find it hard to say no whenever anyone asks me to help	I get really overwhelmed with too much to do and end up working long days without time to wind down
I volunteer to take on responsibilities even if they are not mine		
I constantly remind myself about all the things I should be doing		
I find it hard to delegate		

It's hard to say 'no' to other people's requests even if they are unreasonable		
I often feel over-burdened by other people's demands and expectations		
I feel responsible when anything stops going to plan and blame myself for things others don't even think of		
I can feel irritated or resentful towards people who seem to take advantage of my generosity		
I don't have time to care for my own needs; it is more important to get the job done		

GROWTH skills for 'chronic heroes'

Use your Guide

The first step is to offer thanks and appreciation to your inner hero for their huge efforts. Rather than constantly driving yourself to do more, perhaps your hero is ready for a little well-earned rest and ease! Don't allow values such as responsibility and care for others to dominate or overshadow other values such as self-care, autonomy, choice and self-compassion. Keep a reasonable balance between caring for yourself and for others. Your needs are not in competition with those of others, but instead recognise that both are important alongside one another.

Coping with guilt can involve recognising that feeling conflicted and under pressure is part of the complexity of general practice and doesn't necessarily indicate that you have fallen short or have not done enough in your efforts to live according to your values.

Ready for Action

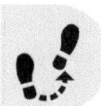

Create some healthy boundaries and prioritise the most important activities. Can you choose actions which move you towards a broader range of values, even if this is uncomfortable or brings up feelings of guilt? Can you let go of the inner demand to live up to impossible or unrealistic standards? Can you delegate, share tasks, or ask for help if you need it? As a first step, perhaps you could support or mentor a colleague to take on a new role or responsibility.

Open and Observe

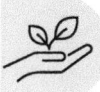

Try to create brief pauses in your day, which may allow you to notice 'chronic hero' beliefs, when they show up. Observe what thoughts, feelings and behavioural urges have shown up. Are there any patterns? Take a breath and try to step back from these emotions and beliefs if they are unhelpful or contributing to your stress. Rather than reacting in autopilot, what might be a more helpful response?

Do you need to check in with your physical body, and pay attention to signals such as 'I'm tired, hungry or thirsty'? Taking time to recognise and act on your personal needs may help you to cope more effectively with pressure and stressful situations.

Wise Mind

Allow your **Wise Mind** to take the lead and make decisions, acknowledging your hero's contribution but not allowing them to take complete control. **Wise Mind** helps you listen to realistic, balanced thoughts rather than buying into self-criticism or beliefs about excessive responsibility. When facing difficulties, our **Wise Mind** recognises that taking all the responsibility and blaming yourself is extreme, unhelpful and unrealistic. Situations are multifactorial, and no one can completely control every outcome.

EXERCISE: Create a responsibility pie chart

If you are wrestling with excessive guilt over a complex situation that may not be entirely your fault, a responsibility pie chart can help you take a more objective and realistic perspective.

First, describe the situation, problem, or event that you are taking responsibility for:

Now, think about who (people) and what (places/organisations/situations) are involved and list them below. You can include yourself, but put yourself last on the list:

Now draw a circle and allocate a slice of the 'pie' to each person or organisation on the list. Think how big a slice of the pie you might allocate, according to how much responsibility and control each individual has for the situation. Draw lines to divide up the pie. Make sure you fit your own slice in last.

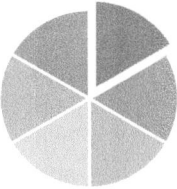

Can you notice any changes in your thoughts and feelings? Does it help to be more aware of other people's responsibility and control alongside your own? What different actions might you take after thinking about the situation like this?

Thrive and Balance and Healthy Life Habits

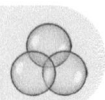

When you are struggling with uncomfortable feelings of guilt, or if something has gone wrong, try to foster self-compassion, saying to yourself: "This is a difficult moment, I'm doing the best that I can right now. I don't have to be perfect". Remember that experiencing guilt may be a sign of being a caring person, rather than indicating that you've done something wrong.

You might also benefit from seeking support from colleagues and friends. Can you create a network of relationships and allow people to support you, rather than always feeling that you need to be 'strong' or to care for others?

Can you let go of any responsibility or duty, perhaps by delegating within your team? You could experiment with using a coaching style of leadership, which encourages others to develop their skills and self-belief. Use any time that you free up to do something that you care about!

And finally, remember to make healthy life choices that balance needs such as physical health, nutrition, hobbies and social life alongside duty and responsibility. What small changes might you try?

Matthew seeks more balance and self-compassion:

"I was feeling completely responsible for caring for my mother's illness, so I drew out at a responsibility pie-chart:

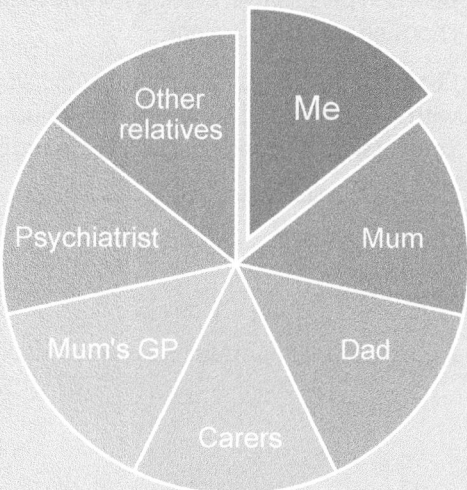

It was really helpful to think about all the other people that have some responsibility for this situation. Before, I was imagining that I was responsible for the whole pie! This has helped me to step back and recognise that I do need to make time and space to look after myself as well – and I know Mum would want me to do this.

I'm going to set some boundaries around my work. I know this will feel uncomfortable, but I will try to be kind and act as my own supportive mentor – using the advice I know that I would give to a colleague in the same situation!

I'm going to make myself a flask of my favourite tea and take it into work – and have a cup when I'm feeling overwhelmed. I will try taking a few mindful sips and use this time as a pause to help me keep myself balanced and not allow my 'chronic hero' to dominate."

Chapter Summary: Personality traits and traps

- Unhealthy perfectionism, obsessional focus, imposter syndrome and being a 'chronic hero' are personality traits which can negatively impact a clinician's wellbeing.

- Working to our strengths allows us to realise our potential and thrive in the face of stress and challenge.

- Coping with perfectionism involves taking small steps to relax unrelenting standards, practising self-compassion, and developing a growth mindset.

- Managing self-doubt in imposter syndrome involves putting imposter beliefs in perspective, looking for evidence of personal success and choosing confident actions.

- Coping with 'chronic hero' traits could involve increasing collaboration with colleagues and engaging with values of self-care and self-compassion, alongside duty and responsibility.

Final thoughts

What are the most important messages for you from this chapter?

Take an action step

What are your next steps? What actions will you take as a result of reading this chapter?

What steps can you take to work to your personal strengths and support any areas of vulnerability?

08 Low mood

- Are you feeling flat, or finding it difficult to enjoy life and see a bright future ahead?

- Is it hard to motivate yourself to get to work or to complete your daily tasks?

- Have you started to withdraw from friends and family or cut down things you used to enjoy, because the effort just seems too great?

- Do you want to learn some evidence-based ways to lift low mood and increase your motivation? Keep reading...

8.1 Recognising low mood

Low mood is common. Sometimes there's an obvious trigger, such as a stressful life event, and at other times it may build up gradually or seem to come from nowhere.

If depressed mood becomes more persistent, you might start to notice a pattern of feeling flat, fed up or demotivated, or have less energy or have difficulty concentrating. You may also experience trouble with sleep and appetite, or just find that life is a bit harder than normal. Low mood can also create agitation, irritability and anger.

In this chapter we will look at ways of overcoming low mood and improving motivation including:

- Identifying meaningful, enjoyable and important activities which are likely to lift your mood and connect you to others

- Setting realistic small goals to increase your enthusiasm and energy

- Using mindfulness and gratitude to unhook from negative thoughts, and to acknowledge and appreciate positive experiences

- Using your **Wise Mind** to make helpful choices about ways to support, encourage and motivate yourself

How is your mood?

Is low mood having a negative impact on your life? If so, it may be time to make some changes or try out some strategies to lift your mood.

Look at the questions below and see how many of these possible signs of low mood you recognise:

Signs of low mood	Tick if you have noticed this:
You have been feeling low for at least a few weeks	
You are more tearful than usual	
You lack motivation and find it harder to start or complete important activities	
You are no longer enjoying things that you used to find interesting or fun	
You are finding it harder to concentrate	
You see yourself negatively and can be self-critical or blame yourself when things go wrong	
You are more irritable and intolerant of others	
You have withdrawn or become isolated from friends and family	
You feel tired and lethargic, which is not improved by rest	
You are starting to think that the future looks bleak and that things may never improve	

If you have ticked more than three or four of these items, then you might need to think more about your mood and consider how much it is affecting you. Keep going with this chapter for some ideas about how to make some changes and improvements.

8.2 **When low mood becomes depression**

It is important to recognise when low mood may start slipping into depression, with persistent or overwhelming feelings of unhappiness, lethargy or irritability. Depression can have a major impact on your life and your ability to function at work and at home. It can also be effectively treated, so it's important to spot it early, and take appropriate action.

Here's a reminder of the common symptoms of depression (NICE, 2022a):

Core symptoms	Associated symptoms
• Feeling down, depressed or hopeless • Loss of interest or pleasure in doing things	• Disturbed sleep • Changes in appetite or weight • Fatigue and loss of energy • Agitation or slowing of movements • Poor concentration or indecisiveness • Feelings of worthlessness or guilt • Suicidal thoughts or acts

You also might wish to use a validated assessment tool, such as PHQ9, or the Hospital Anxiety and Depression Scale (HADS) to assess your depression scores.

Thoughts of suicide

When you feel low or depressed, you may experience thoughts of suicide or self-harm, or of not wanting to continue living. Having these thoughts does not mean that you will act on them, and they will often pass as your mood starts to lift again.

However, having thoughts about harming yourself is an important sign that you need support, so it's extremely important to seek help and advice. Talking about suicidal thoughts will not make you more likely to act on them, and sharing how you are feeling might help you find better ways to cope with difficult emotions.

When to seek help

If you think you may be experiencing depression, or you are experiencing suicidal thoughts, we strongly recommend that you seek help from your GP, your local mental health team, or a national support service such as Practitioner Health.

Support is available and can make a huge difference, enabling you to take the first steps towards recovery and wellbeing.

Heather, GP Partner: *"I've been feeling low for a few months now. I have noticed that I'm getting slower at work, and lately I've been finding it almost impossible to get through all my tasks by the end of the day. I started working on my day off, but I'm still struggling to keep up. I had a complaint from a patient where I didn't complete her insurance report in time, and that really knocked my confidence. There's a lot going on at home as well. My mother-in-law has been poorly and that puts extra strain on my husband, and we have been arguing a lot. I have a teenage daughter who is stressed and anxious about her upcoming GCSEs and that affects us all.*

I have started feeling very flat and low. I'm constantly tired and I just can't seem to motivate myself to do any of the activities that I used to. I'm just about

> coping at work, but I know that I'm not very efficient and my concentration and focus is nowhere near as good as before. I feel stuck, and I have no idea what to do to make things any better."

8.3 What are the causes of low mood?

In the next section we will look at some things which may trigger low mood.

Life stresses and problems

Life stresses and pressures can be a catalyst for, or exacerbate low mood. Look at the following list and put a tick by any that are affecting you at the moment:

Stressful life event or situation	Tick if this is affecting you:
Problems or stress at work	
Relationship difficulties with a spouse or partner	
Other family problems or challenges	
Financial problems	
Health problems (affecting you or a loved one)	
Bereavement and loss	
Coping with a complaint or performance procedures	
Fears or worries about the future, e.g. retirement planning	
Pressure to achieve (e.g. exams or other targets)	
Any kind of physical, emotional or sexual abuse	
Arguments or disagreements with friends or family	
Anything else important?	

Coping with life stresses and problems

It's common to feel low when coping with multiple life stresses, but if you start to feel overwhelmed or you are starting to see your problems as impossible to solve, this can have a negative impact on your mood. An alternative is starting to believe that you can cope with the problems that life throws at you. This can help to build your confidence and help to lift your mood. We talk more about this in *Chapter 11.*

8.4 Different responses to the same situation

Let's explore how different people might respond to work challenges in different ways, leading to different emotions and behaviours:

A patient complains...
You receive a note in your tray asking you to speak to the practice manager about a patient who has complained that you were running very late to see them last week. How might you react?

Thoughts	The practice manager must think I'm completely incompetent. I'm such a useless doctor...	Oh no – this is a disaster! It will turn into a major complaint. What if I'm struck off?	This person is completely unreasonable! How dare they complain when I put in so much effort?	Oh no, this is not very pleasant. I remember the day and there was an emergency that made me very late. I will explain to the practice manager, I'm sure she will understand...
Feelings	Sad, demoralised	Anxious	Angry, annoyed	Calm, thoughtful
In the body	Tired, headache	Agitated, pacing	Tense	Relaxed
Behaviour	Go back to my room and try to avoid seeing the practice manager because I feel ashamed and embarrassed.	Rush to the practice manager's room seeking reassurance that everything will be OK.	Storm into the practice manager's office and let off steam about the ungrateful patient. Irritable and snappy with colleagues.	Take a breath and then go and talk to the practice manager. Explain the circumstances and ask for her advice about writing back to the patient.
Impact of these actions	Feel more isolated, lonely and fed up. No opportunity to talk through or resolve the problem.	Loss of confidence in abilities at work.	Increase in anger and strained relationships with colleagues.	Gain support with how to cope with the problem effectively.

Ask yourself this: If you were facing a similar situation:

How would you interpret the situation – what thoughts would you have about it?	
How might these thoughts affect how you feel?	
What might you notice in your body?	
What would you do?	
What would be the impact of these actions? How might these actions affect your feelings? Would they be helpful or unhelpful?	

The cycle of low mood

When you feel low and fed up, you may also begin to view the world in a more negative way and behave in unhelpful ways that worsen your mood even more. A CBT framework (see figure below) can be a helpful way to explore how low mood affects you.

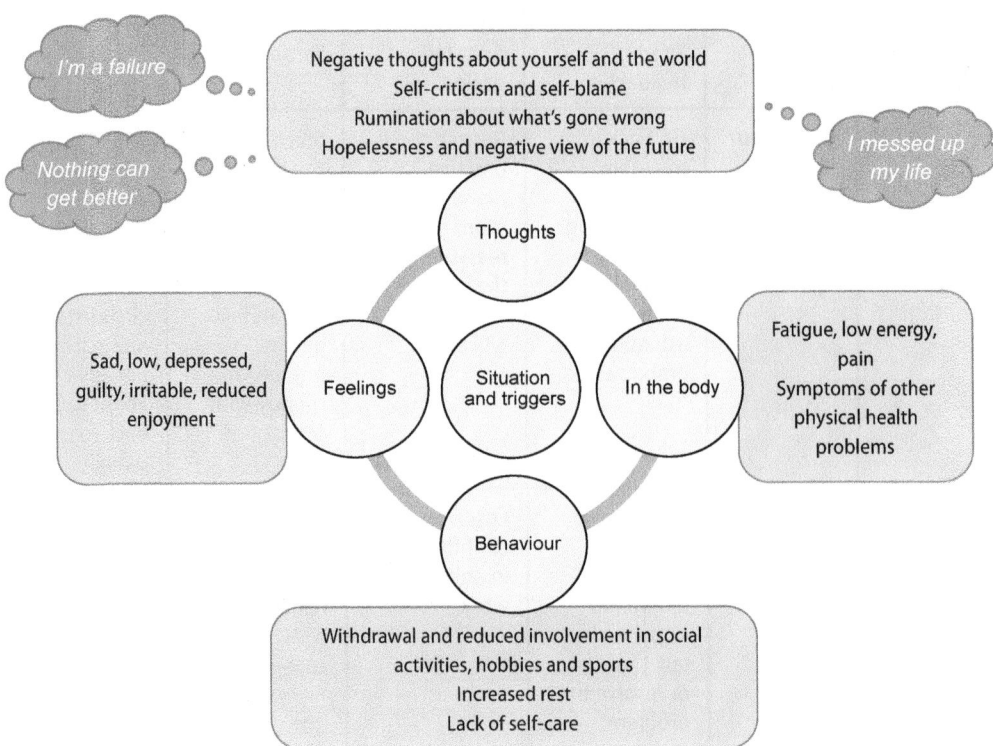

PAUSE AND REFLECT: CBT framework for low mood

Can you notice any patterns or reactions of thinking patterns, emotions, physical reactions or behaviour that suggest you are struggling with low mood? Complete the following table:

Aspect of low mood	What examples have you noticed?
Negative thinking: lack of motivation and pessimistic or critical thoughts about yourself, the world or the future	
Feelings such as low mood, lack of enjoyment, irritability	
In the body: physical reactions such as fatigue, lethargy, pain or sleep problems	
Behaviour: withdrawal from others, reduced participation in activities or hobbies, reduced self-care	

Heather reflects: *"I have noticed a lot of changes that suggest my mood is low. It's only when I stop and look back that I realise how far I've slipped down compared to when I'm at my best."*

Aspect of low mood	Heather's examples
Negative thinking: lack of motivation and pessimistic or critical thoughts about yourself, the world or the future	I'm struggling a lot with motivation. I have lots of negative thoughts about how useless I am. I would never harm myself, but it feels hard to imagine how anything can get any better.
Feelings such as low mood, lack of enjoyment, irritability	I feel guilty and ashamed that I'm not doing many things that I know are important. My mood is flat, and nothing seems enjoyable. I'm much more irritable with my family.
In the body: physical reactions such as fatigue, lethargy, pain or sleep problems	I feel tired and have a lot of headaches. My sleep is poor – I find it hard to drop off or I find myself awake in the night.

Behaviour: withdrawal from others, reduced participation in activities or hobbies, reduced self-care	I'm just about managing at work, but I have cut down nearly all of the things I used to do for fun. I don't feel bothered to do almost anything. I don't have the energy to see friends and I'm avoiding phone calls from my sister.

Stuck in the low mood 'swamp'

Feeling low can make you feel like you are stuck in a giant muddy swamp. Life feels extremely difficult, and your surroundings are grim. Your body feels fatigued and even the smallest step is a huge effort.

You may start to believe that there's no way out and that nothing will help. You feel hopeless and you have a barrage of negative thoughts as your mind tells you, "What's the point? I'm too tired, I won't enjoy anything, and I can't achieve much anyway!" So, you cut down your usual activities, which seem pointless and exhausting.

You stand still in the swamp, giving up on trying to get anywhere and allow yourself to sink into the heavy, dark mud around you...

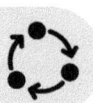

The vicious cycle of reducing activity

Sinking into the low mood swamp tends to involve reducing enjoyable, meaningful and social activities. This is because a depressed or flat mood, lack of motivation, fatigue and concentration problems all make it harder to engage and enjoy activities as usual.

We may also become irritable and snappy, comfort eat, or spend long hours mindlessly scrolling our phone or using social media. These actions may temporarily numb or distance us from difficult feelings, but often lead to increased negative feelings over time.

In the short term, doing less might feel like a necessary choice because you are feeling so tired and fed up. But doing fewer activities means that you are missing out on opportunities to do things that you care about. You lose the chance to engage your Drive system and boost your confidence by achieving your goals. As a consequence, life starts to feel even more meaningless and flat, and your mood drops still further.

So, you slip into a vicious cycle of reducing activity, which makes you feel even more depressed and low:

```
                    ┌─────────────────────────┐
                    │        Thoughts         │
                    │       I'm useless       │
                    │      I'm a failure      │
                    │  I can't do anything right│
                    └─────────────────────────┘

┌─────────────────────────┐         ┌─────────────────────────┐
│        Behaviour        │         │       In the body       │
│  Cut down activities, social │    │     Fatigue, aches      │
│        withdrawal       │         │                         │
└─────────────────────────┘         └─────────────────────────┘

                    ┌─────────────────────────┐
                    │        Feelings         │
                    │     Low, flat, sad,     │
                    │        irritable        │
                    └─────────────────────────┘
```

8.5 The route out of the swamp

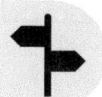

One of the best ways to get out of the low mood swamp is to start walking really slowly and take very small steps. This involves getting **Ready for Action** by 'behaving as if...' you feel slightly better.

Using behavioural activation (Martell *et al.*, 2001) to increase activity is an evidence-based strategy which has been shown to be as effective as CBT for treating depression (Uphoff *et al.*, 2020).

This involves planning to do just a little more activity, based on following your inner **Guide**, even if you are experiencing low mood, fatigue and negative thoughts. Your mind may tell you "I can't be bothered, this won't help, and I'm just too tired to try...". However, it's often more helpful to make decisions about activity based on what's important and meaningful to you, rather than based on enjoyment or motivation. And you can plan small changes that are realistic and achievable.

Increasing valued activities often leads to a gradual increase in energy and an improved sense of achievement, and helps to lift low mood. It may take time to notice these effects. But eventually, as you keep walking, and keep participating in meaningful activities, you might find that you have reached firmer ground. Your steps start to feel easier, and your surroundings are nicer. Your mood is brighter, and you are able to look up and spot an amazing view – you have made it out of the low mood swamp!

Choosing activities

There are no absolute rules for the choice of activities for behavioural activation, although connecting with people socially and physical activity are both particularly effective for improving low mood.

It's often helpful to ask your inner **Guide** about the people and activities that matter most to you. Use the following table to help you reflect on what activities might be important or meaningful for you:

Who and what is most important to you? What activities are related to these important parts of your life?	
What are your core values? What kind of person would you choose to be – at work and in your personal life?	
Imagine you could wave a magic wand and feel motivated, enthusiastic and happy tomorrow. How would this affect how you spent the day? What would you do?	
What activities did you used to enjoy or do regularly in the past?	

Here are Heather's answers:

Who and what is most important to you? What activities are related to these important parts of your life?	My family really matter – I want to support my daughter with her anxiety, and to improve my relationship with my husband. And actually, I matter too. I think I've lost sight of looking after myself alongside all my other responsibilities.
What are your core values? What kind of person would you choose to be – at work and in your personal life?	My core values are around care and aspiration. I want to get back to being more efficient and professional, and have enough energy to support everyone I care about at home.
Imagine you could wave a magic wand and feel motivated, enthusiastic and happy tomorrow. How would this affect how you spent the day? What would you do?	If I felt better, I would probably take a day out and spend it doing something enjoyable with my family. Maybe we would go for a family walk or have a pub lunch together.
What activities did you used to enjoy or do regularly in the past?	I used to have a good habit of going to the gym several times a week and I enjoyed feeling a bit fitter.

Balancing activities

Try to make sure that your activities are varied and bring some SPICE to your day or week! Ideally, this means that activities should involve one of the following:

- **S**uccess or achievement
- **P**hysical activity and moving your body
- **I**mportant and meaningful to you
- **C**onnection or closeness to others
- **E**njoyable, relaxing and fun

The following table includes some examples of different types of SPICE activities. Make a note of any ideas that you might try.

Type of activity	Examples	What could you try?
Success or achievement	Try a new recipe – or an old favourite Learn something new, e.g. touch-typing or photography Do the laundry or some DIY Tidy up one room of your house Start your tax return Tick one easy item off your to-do list Clear your email inbox	
Physical activity	Take your dog for a walk Do a 10 minute online workout Dance to one song Go for a hike, a bike ride or a jog Swim in a pool or outdoors Do yoga or Pilates Bounce on a trampoline Do strength training Play a sport such as football, tennis or golf Mow the lawn or do some gardening	
Important or meaningful	Do some online education Make a start with your appraisal or e-portfolio Start a podcast or a blog Volunteer for a local charity Go shopping for an elderly relative Update your CV or apply for a job Make a business plan for a new venture Book a dentist appointment	

Connection or closeness	Join a book group or choir Give or receive a massage Play a board game, or plan a film night or quiz with friends or family Stroke your pet Email, message or call a friend Tell someone a joke Create a slideshow of your favourite photos	
Enjoyable, relaxing or fun	Play an instrument or listen to music Do a jigsaw or mindful colouring Knitting, sewing, art or creative writing Go to the cinema, theatre or ballet Practise mindfulness Have a home spa session Do a virtual escape room Go to the hairdresser Put on make-up or your favourite outfit Take a long shower or bubble bath Watch a comedy	

Keep the steps small

What's your reaction to the above list? Does it make you feel motivated and enthused to get going? Or is there a sense of pressure, overload or fatigue, which makes it hard to get started?

As we learnt in *Chapter 7*, it's common for health professionals to have high standards and a tendency towards perfectionism. This helps us achieve a huge amount but can be a barrier to getting started when we are recovering from depressed mood.

Rather than giving up completely, you can build your confidence by planning small, **micro-steps** towards change. We first met these in *Chapter 2* on being **Ready for Action**. Ideally, they take only from 2 to 10 minutes to complete.

Micro-steps involve tiny changes, which are often so small that you think they won't make much difference. They are not designed to solve a major problem but are a tiny step in that direction. They help to break ingrained habits and act as a reminder that you can make choices about what you do each day. They can get you started on the path to change and create a ripple effect that leads to improvements over time.

Examples of micro-steps include:

- Walking around the car park for 5 minutes at lunchtime to get some fresh air
- Sending a text message to an old friend

- Picking out an outfit to wear that you used to love
- Finding your trainers and putting them by the front door.

EXERCISE: Planning micro-steps

Choose a life area and then plan a micro-step that moves you in this direction:

Planning micro-steps	Example	Complete your answers below
Choose a value or life area that matters to you	Family life and getting a balance between work and personal life	
What's one tiny step that moves you in this direction?	On Sunday I will play a board game with my family	
How long will the activity take? Aim for 5 minutes or less. Even 1 minute will help you get started!	If we choose a quick game it will only take around 10–15 minutes	
How confident are you that you will do this? 1 = not confident at all 2 = a little confident 3 = so-so 4 = fairly confident 5 = I will do it! Aim for a rating of 4 or 5	3 – we might get caught up in other things and not get around to it. My kids may not be very enthusiastic.	
If your confidence rating is less than 4 or 5, what can you do to help? For example: Lower the bar: make the goal easier or shorter Ask for help from someone Think about something you have achieved in the past to boost your confidence	I will ask my husband to help me remember. I could also try to involve the kids by asking them in advance what they would like to play.	
What's the next small step towards your goal?	I could plan some one-to-one time with my daughter. We could go for a walk or go shopping together	

8.6 Activity diary

To keep track of your activities and mood, you might find it helpful to complete an activity diary. It can be helpful to do this for around two weeks, covering both your working days and days away from work. What patterns can you notice?

Time	What was the activity? How long did you do it for?	Was this activity linked to SPICE? **S**uccess or achievement **P**hysical activity or movement **I**mportant or meaningful **C**onnection or closeness **E**njoyment or fun	How was your mood after doing this (1–10)?
6am			
7am			
8am			
9am			
10am			
11am			
12 noon			
1pm			
2pm			
3pm			
4pm			
5pm			
6pm			
7pm			
8pm			
9pm			
10pm			
11pm			

Learning from your experiences

After completing an activity diary for low mood, it can also be helpful to reflect on any patterns of activity and mood. Ask yourself:

- What can you notice about how you spend your time?

- Are there any links between your activities and your mood?

- Do any activities lead to a dip or lowering in your mood?

- Do any activities seem to boost or lift your mood?

- How might this information change how you choose to spend your time each day?

8.7 Keeping it going

Once you have made some changes to your life and hopefully started to feel a bit brighter, the next step is planning how to keep things going and avoid slipping back into the low mood swamp. Here are some tips for keeping up your positive habits.

Structure and routine

Creating a routine can help you stick to helpful activities that will keep up a more positive mood over time. As your new patterns of activity turn into habits, it becomes easier to do them. Make sure your routine is flexible and can adapt to any new situations or events. We talk more about ways to create healthy life habits in *Chapter 6*.

Write it down

Keeping a record of your activity levels using your phone, a diary or planner will help you to keep track of your achievements and can motivate you to continue making new changes.

Take some time each week to look through your diary and check how you are getting on. This will help to keep you on the right track.

Seek help and support

Think about who could help or support you in planning and carrying out any of these changes, including friends, family, pets, your phone, your diary or an online community.

8.8 Managing negative thinking

In this next section, we will look at some of the negative thoughts and thinking styles that may sometimes keep you stuck in the low mood swamp.

Negative visitors to our mind

When we are feeling low, we often take on a more negative view of ourselves and the world. We can only see half the picture, which tends to have a negative bias or filter colouring our perception of situations. These thoughts can be like a repetitive treadmill, as we ruminate about the same recriminations, self-blame and worry thoughts over and over again.

It's as if our mind is having a number of gloomy and pessimistic visitors, who don't want to leave! This is similar to the idea of the negative patients who visit the surgery that we discussed in *Chapter 4*.

So who are these negative visitors that might pay your mind a visit when you are feeling low? Perhaps you are familiar with some of the following characters:

The pessimist – who keeps telling you that life has gone completely wrong, and there's no hope of improvement

> Nothing's going to work out well. What's the point in trying?

The hyper-critic – giving you a hard time and being critical of every small mistake

> You're such an idiot – why didn't you do a better job?

The worn-out and weary – reminding you how tired you are and how you just don't have energy to get anything done

> I'm just too exhausted to do anything more...

The blamer – unfairly blaming you for everything that goes wrong

> It's all your fault – you should have done a better job...

The motivation mugger – expects the worst and encourages you to give up and stop trying

> You'll have a terrible time if you go out with your friends. Just give up and stay home alone...

PAUSE AND REFLECT: The impact of negative mind visitors

Do you recognise any of these negative visitors and how they see the world?

What effect do they have on your mood and on your actions?

Make a note of your thoughts here:

Coping with negative thoughts

So how can you cope when these negative visitors and their unhelpful way of viewing the world show up in your mind?

Start by observing and noticing when these negative characters have shown up. This allows you to create a little bit of distance and perspective between your **Wise Mind** and these visitors with their gloomy messages.

As you create some space between you and the negative thoughts, you may begin to remember that these thoughts are not facts. You don't need to listen to these characters or believe the unhelpful things they are saying to you.

A Wise alternative view

The next step is to use the perspective of your **Wise Mind**. What would a supportive coach, mentor, colleague or best friend tell you? What advice would you offer to others? What is the whole picture rather than the filtered view through the negative lens of low mood?

Your **Wise Mind** can recognise when the negative visitors have come to call but doesn't automatically buy into their point of view. It responds to the negative visitors with assertiveness, fairness and kindness, rather than arguing, criticising or blaming them. Your Wise Mind believes that you are capable of dealing with the problems that you face, and gives caring and sensible advice about different ways to approach the situation.

Ask yourself:

- What supportive or encouraging message would your **Wise Mind** give you when the negative visitors have come to call?

- What advice would your **Wise Mind** give you? What Wise action could you take?

- How can you use your **Wise Mind** to help when you are starting to feel low?

Make a note of your answers here:

Sinking into rumination

Do you ever get stuck in rumination, where you repeatedly think back over something that's gone wrong? This is a bit like getting stuck in the low mood swamp, and these persistent negative thoughts are also usually accompanied by low energy and a lack of motivation to break free. You might get stuck in loops of negative thoughts such as:

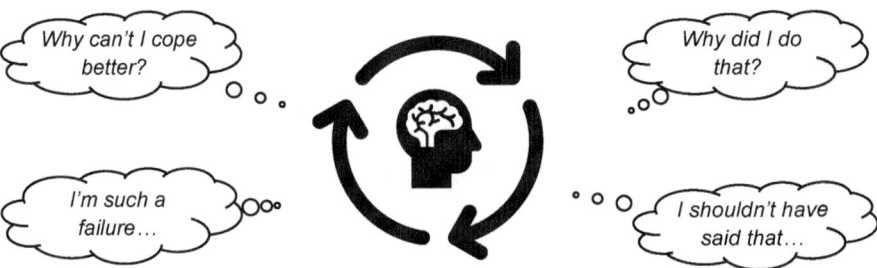

Here are some steps you could try to break away from repetitive rumination in low mood:

Stepping out of rumination	How can you use this? What will you try?
Open and Observe Start to notice when you've got stuck in a negative thinking loop. Use your five senses or 'notice and name' your thoughts and feelings. Put the thoughts in a revolving door rather than allowing them to stick. Then move on to a SPICE activity with your full attention.	
Use distraction It's easy to slip into rumination when you have less to do, are on your own or unoccupied. What activities could you use to shift your energy and attention away from negative thoughts and towards something meaningful or important?	
Be kind to yourself Many of the negative visitors in low mood involve self-criticism and self-blame. Instead, can you be a little kinder to yourself? How might you demonstrate some self-compassion and acceptance?	

Write it down Journaling or keeping a diary of your thoughts and feelings may help to sort out what's going through your mind and make your inner experiences clearer and less overwhelming.	
Problem-solving If negative thoughts relate to a particular problem, it can be helpful to use problem-solving to find ways to cope with it. We talk more about this in *Chapter 5*.	
Seek support Sharing your experiences with others may help you feel more connected and less alone. Try talking to a friend, colleague, family member, your own GP, or a counsellor or therapist.	

 ## *Gratitude and appreciation*

To balance the tendency to slip into negative thinking, we can also actively pay attention to any small positive life experiences, or things that have gone well, rather than only focusing on what's gone wrong. Taking time to do this each day can help to counteract the negative visitors and their gloomy way of looking at the world.

Seek gratitude and appreciation	Example	What can you think of?
What do you appreciate right now, on this day or this moment? It can be tiny, like someone smiling at you, the sunlight through the trees, or your favourite soft cushion. Look around and make a note of at least three things.	The sun is shining, and the sky looks beautiful. I enjoyed my morning coffee. My colleague smiled when she saw me today and asked about my weekend	
Consider keeping a gratitude journal or diary, where you make a note each day about one or two small things that you appreciate or feel pleased and proud of.	I had a compliment from one of the reception staff about my new haircut! A patient thanked me for listening	

Heather decided to put into action on a regular basis some activities that were starting to lift her mood. She recognised that her family and work were the most important things in her life, but nothing could change unless she looked after her own needs as well. She set an intention to create more balance and to involve her family more in both her leisure and also in creating some time for herself.

"Now I go to the gym for an hour on Saturday mornings, and I can listen to my favourite podcasts uninterrupted! When my 'worn out and weary' or 'critic' mind visitors pop up, I notice them and then picture them going back out of a revolving door. My Wise Mind often reminds me to 'share the load' so I'm trying to talk more to my husband and my partners at work and to ask for help when needed.

We've made a family habit to share some of the household chores, and my daughter cooks with me once a week so we have time to chat. At weekends, we take it in turns to plan a family activity, and I try to schedule some time with my husband at least once a month where we go for a meal or to the cinema. Things definitely feel better and I'm keen to keep these changes going as a positive routine."

Chapter summary: Low mood

- Overcoming low mood and lack of motivation involves taking small action steps.

- When stuck in the low mood swamp we feel exhausted and lose enjoyment and motivation, but cutting down important and meaningful activities usually often worsens depressed mood as a vicious cycle.

- Getting out of the swamp involves taking small steps and behaving 'as if' you feel better, which gradually increases energy and lifts low mood.

- SPICE activities involve: Success or achievement, Physical activity, Important and meaningful, Connection or closeness, Enjoyable, relaxing and fun.

- Making change through micro-steps will be more manageable and prevent overwhelm.

- Finding gratitude and appreciation for small positive experiences can shift your focus out of gloomy thoughts and lift your mood.

Final thoughts

What are the most important messages for you from this chapter?

Take an action step

What are your next steps? What actions will you take as a result of reading this chapter?

Are there any regular actions or patterns of behaviour that you might try to practise or develop to lift low mood?

09 Anxiety and uncertainty

- Do you often feel tense, on edge, nervous or irritable or find it difficult to wind down and relax after work?

- Is your mind frequently in a whir of worry as you catastrophise and imagine the worst possible scenarios?

- Do you hate taking risks and struggle to manage the uncertainty and unpredictability of working in primary care?

- Do you want to be less troubled by anxiety and mental preoccupation? Keep reading…

9.1 What is anxiety?

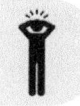

Anxiety is a normal human reaction to anything that seems scary or threatening. It is an autonomic response arising from the sympathetic nervous system, which can be triggered by a wide range of stressful events, situations or decisions. Experiencing a distressing or traumatic experience can also lead to anxiety about having to face a similar situation again.

Triggering the anxiety response leads to:

- Feelings of fear, anxiety, nervousness and unease

- Changes in the body causing physiological symptoms of anxiety

- Negative thoughts such as catastrophising and focusing on the worst possible outcomes, or not trusting yourself to cope if things go wrong

- Changes in behaviour to try to keep yourself safe such as avoidance, asking for reassurance, or trying to reduce the risk by checking or worrying.

The pressures of living and working in the inherently uncertain environment of primary care can also make us anxious. When we find it hard to tolerate uncertainty, we may experience a deluge of worries about potential problems and risks such as making a mistake, missing something important, or receiving a complaint. These fears may be accurate and factual, but they may also become exaggerated or involve consequences that are objectively unlikely to take place or are outside our control.

Anxiety can also lead to a range of behaviours that have a detrimental effect on our efficiency at work, as well as on our wellbeing and relationships. We may use excessive planning and preparation, or repeated reassurance-seeking and checking as a way of avoiding or eliminating uncertainty. These actions often have a negative impact, making it harder to get through our mounting workload, or to switch off afterwards.

Despite the bad press, anxiety is not all bad. The nervousness and fear that arise before sitting an exam or giving a presentation can keep your mind focused, encourage you to prepare, and help you to perform on the day. Being aware of possible negative clinical outcomes can help us to maintain high standards and work safely within our competence. So, the aim is not to eliminate anxiety altogether, but to make sure it stays in balance, and doesn't become overwhelming or get in the way of living our lives.

In this chapter we will learn more about how to cope with anxiety and uncertainty. This includes:

- Following your inner **Guide** towards what's important and not allowing anxiety or worry to pull you away from the things that you value

- Building your confidence by taking small steps towards important activities that you may be avoiding or putting off

- Finding ways to create some space and step back from uncomfortable thoughts, worries, feelings and sensations of anxiety

- Seeking a wider perspective and making Wise choices and decisions rather than allowing your anxious mind to take control.

9.2 Are you struggling with anxiety?

The first step is to recognise if you are living with excessive anxiety that limits or affects your life and relationships. Take a look at the following checklist. If you recognise more than three or four possible signs, this may mean that you would benefit from developing some new strategies and skills in coping with anxiety.

Possible signs of anxiety	Tick if you recognise this
Do you often worry about things before they happen?	
Do you find it difficult to relax and wind down or switch off worries in your mind?	
Do you suffer frequent physical complaints such as abdominal pain, headaches or muscle pains?	

Do you often try to avoid situations that are likely to make you feel anxious or worried?	
Do you frequently ask for reassurance from others?	
Do you often double- or triple-check to ensure that you have done something correctly?	
Do worries or a racing mind often affect your sleep?	
Do you often feel afraid that something really bad might happen?	
Do you seem to worry or get anxious more than friends, family or colleagues?	

Paola, newly qualified GP Partner: *"I've always been quite an anxious person and I don't really like taking risks – I prefer to know that everything has been done properly. Sometimes I find myself checking or repeating tasks a few times until I'm certain it's been done right. Things were OK when I was training. I was a little prone to getting anxious and a bit slower than the other trainees, but I was able to complete the programme without major problems.*

Once I qualified as a GP, my husband and I decided to change area and move closer to our families. I was offered a partnership in a large practice, and I took it on despite some reservations.

The way the practice works is very different from my training practice. There's a lot less interaction and support. The GPs used to ask each other questions and for advice, but since Covid everyone works a lot more independently and often from home. When I feel unsure, I often don't have anyone to ask, and this makes me feel really anxious. I've started double- and triple-checking my notes and results, and I often go back over a surgery afterwards to make sure I haven't missed anything. This makes it very hard to leave on time.

I'm not focused at home either. I'm jittery, edgy and irritable the whole time. My mind is often elsewhere, and I've let my husband take over most of the play and fun with our children. I just get the household chores done and then go to bed."

9.3 Why do we have anxiety?

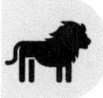

The purpose of anxiety is to help your body rapidly prepare and react to any potential threat or danger. It involves the fight, flight or freeze response that we looked at in *Section 3.7*. This system developed as a survival mechanism to cope with physical danger such as being threatened by a wild animal. To do this, we would have to *fight* off anything that's threatening, take *flight* and move quickly to escape a dangerous situation, or *freeze* so that the prey doesn't notice you or loses interest.

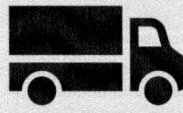 Imagine you are walking across a road that's usually very quiet with hardly any traffic. Suddenly, around the corner veers a huge truck. You realise that it's not slowing down! The driver beeps his horn, and you can hear the roar of the engine.

Without thinking, you start running towards the pavement, and after a few steps, you reach safety as the truck thunders past.

What sensations might you feel in your body?

The fight, flight or freeze response is activated by the sympathetic nervous system, which triggers the release of adrenaline. This affects many different systems of the body, leading to a range of physiological responses to anxiety (see figure below).

This automatic response enables us to run quickly to the side of the road and escape being knocked down by the truck – it ensures survival. But the surge of hormones can be intense and cause unpleasant sensations such as breathlessness, palpitations, nausea and dizziness. And you may even start to worry there is a more serious cause for such marked or distressing symptoms.

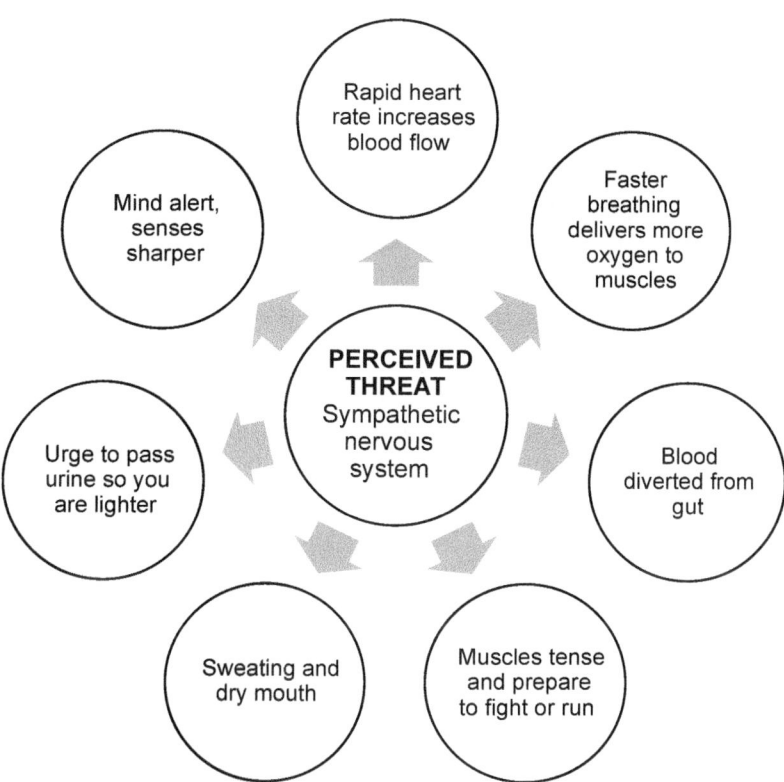

9.4 Anxiety is not dangerous!

The human's brain's incredible capacity to think and imagine gives us the ability to dream, and cope with complex problems. But this can also cause challenges. As we learnt when we looked at the Threat system (*Section 5.6*), the anxiety system will respond in exactly the same way to dangers that are in the real world, as to those that we have imagined or predicted. So, we can have a strong physiological response to worry about imagined fears and future catastrophes, even if these have not yet taken place, or if they are highly unlikely to ever happen.

It is often helpful to remind ourselves and our patients that the physiological responses to anxiety that arise when our sympathetic nervous system is triggered can be very unpleasant but are not dangerous. They are normal reactions to threat that help keep us safe and will gradually fade away once the threat has passed.

It can be helpful to think of anxiety as acting like an alarm system, such as a smoke alarm:

The anxiety alarm system

 Anxiety is an important system that helps keep you safe from possible danger, a bit like a smoke alarm. If there is a fire, you want the alarm to alert you early, so that you can quickly take action to put it out.

It's helpful to have an anxiety response that's roughly in proportion to the threat, so you can trust it to alert you to problems when you need it. But it's less helpful if the anxiety alarm is triggered too easily, perhaps even when there isn't any serious danger.

This is like having a super-sensitive smoke alarm that goes off as soon as your toast starts to brown, but well before it is burning! This can happen when we over-estimate or exaggerate the risks in our mind. We mentioned this in *Chapter 5* when we looked at the importance of balancing the emotion systems.

Sometimes the anxiety response doesn't quickly resolve after the danger has passed, so you may find it hard to stop feeling anxious or worrying. This is like an alarm that's hard to turn off once it starts beeping!

But we don't throw a smoke alarm in the bin if it goes off unnecessarily, because one day there might be a fire and we want to be prepared for this. Likewise, we can't eliminate our anxiety response. But you can learn to recognise feelings of anxiety, quickly check for danger, and learn ways to switch off the alarm and continue with your day, without letting it affect you for too long.

PAUSE AND REFLECT: Noticing your anxiety alarm

- How sensitive is your anxiety alarm? Does it go off more often than is really needed?
- What sort of situations, people and places often set off your alarm system?
- How easy is it to switch it off again?

9.5 Anxiety mind visitors

When facing a situation involving uncertainty or risk, you might notice that many of the negative visitors to your mind that we introduced in *Chapter 4* will rapidly appear, causing feelings of anxiety, worry and panic.

As before, we can think of these as being like anxious patients who come to see us at the surgery. They usually take a very negative view of the world and will tend to:

- **Exaggerate the risks:** they assume the worst possible outcomes are more likely or more serious than they really are. Every headache is a possible brain tumour!

- **Focus on what could go wrong:** they tend to pay more attention to what might go wrong and ignore what might go well.

- **Go round and round:** anxiety visitors are often very persistent and will keep coming back to see you about the same problem over and over again. When these are thoughts that keep popping up in your mind it can be very distracting and make it hard to focus on anything else.

- **Insist that they (and you) can't cope:** anxiety visitors view the world as an extremely risky and dangerous place and will often demand that you need to take exceptional precautions to stay safe. This message can undermine your confidence, and you may begin to feel overwhelmed and avoid challenges.

- **Demand that you try to keep them safe:** anxiety visitors will often insist that you carry out actions that make them feel safer. This is like a patient who wants 'just one more scan or referral to a specialist' for reassurance, or who has spent hours searching the internet for the cause of their symptoms, only to discover all kinds of terrifying new possibilities and scary diagnoses. Going along with their demands might keep the anxiety mind visitors happy in the short term, but it is rarely a lasting solution. They are usually soon back again, demanding further reassurance and certainty that all will be well.

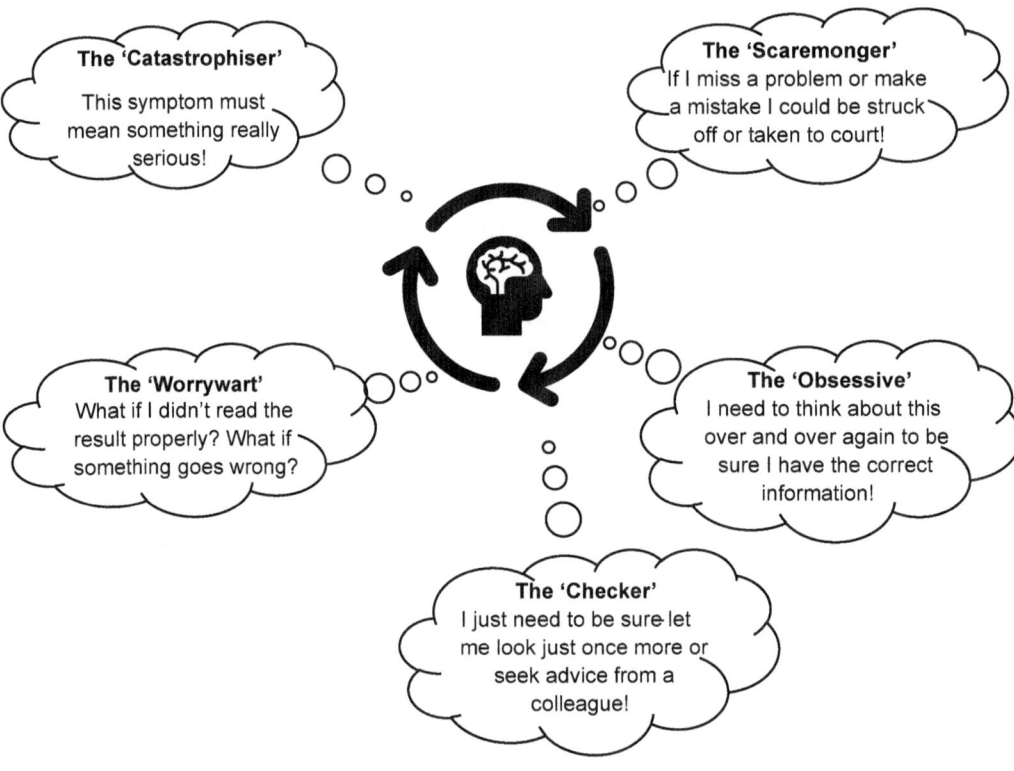

The 'Catastrophiser'

This symptom must mean something really serious!

The 'Scaremonger'
If I miss a problem or make a mistake I could be struck off or taken to court!

The 'Worrywart'
What if I didn't read the result properly? What if something goes wrong?

The 'Obsessive'
I need to think about this over and over again to be sure I have the correct information!

The 'Checker'
I just need to be sure-let me look just once more or seek advice from a colleague!

PAUSE AND REFLECT: Noticing your anxiety mind visitors

- Do unwanted anxiety visitors often show up in your mind? Which ones are most likely to pay you a visit?

- How do you react? Do you argue with them or believe what they say?

- What actions do you take because of their negative messages? Do you avoid any risky situations to keep them quiet? Or do you find yourself asking for reassurance or checking more than is helpful?

- What impact are these unwelcome (and frankly untruthful) visitors having on your life?

Later in the chapter we will look at some strategies to cope when the anxiety visitors show up.

9.6 Anxiety and Away actions

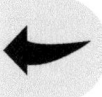

When caught up in loops of worry, you may find yourself repeatedly carrying out Away actions. These are aimed at reducing or preventing feelings of anxiety and worry, but have the added downside of moving you away from important values.

As a clinician you might find yourself avoiding challenges, or people, places and situations that make you feel anxious, and procrastinating or putting off getting started with important activities.

You might also do things to make yourself feel safer, such as asking for reassurance from friends and family, repeated checking or looking for information about a particular topic you are concerned about.

These reactions might help you feel less anxious in the moment, but what's their impact in the long term?

Unfortunately, these are usually Away actions that move you away from your inner **Guide** and from doing the things that you care about. They also tend to undermine your confidence and create a negative spiral of increasing anxiety over time.

Paola, newly qualified GP Partner: *"I can really relate to the anxiety mind visitors – I think they all pay me a visit whenever I start to feel anxious! And I can see that they influence my behaviour too.*

Whenever I feel unsure or there is some kind of uncertainty, I find that the 'Catastrophiser' and the 'Scaremonger' are both very quick to appear! And then I get stuck with the 'Obsessive' and 'Checker', which makes me really slow as I have to go over my work so many times.

I have got stuck in quite a few Away actions where I'm trying to feel less anxious – I often think about work at home or check my emails late at night. But I always feel worse afterwards because there is usually something stressful or an extra piece of work in my inbox. This reminds me of patients who keep Googling their symptoms and then feel more anxious afterwards!"

9.7 Uncertainty in primary care

Managing uncertainty is an inherent aspect of the challenge and emotional demand that can arise from working in primary care. Making a diagnosis in general practice is dynamic and complex. Many patients present with undifferentiated and complex problems, or early in the illness before typical features may have developed. Factors such as multimorbidity and cultural influences can influence the interpretation and presentation of different symptoms. It can be challenging to differentiate between self-limiting conditions and those which may have serious consequences if they go unrecognised. Diagnostic tests themselves are fallible, and balancing risks and benefits can be very difficult.

Coping with uncertainty presents a major challenge but is an essential skill to manage our wellbeing and cope with the pressures of working life. The risks and consequences of medical errors or misdiagnosis are very high, both for the patient and the clinician. However, it's impossible to eliminate or completely avoid uncertainty. We can never be 100% sure what will happen in the future or be certain that nothing will go wrong.

When clinicians struggle to tolerate uncertainty, we may start to experience feelings of anxiety, distress and guilt, and are at greater risk of developing anxiety, work-related stress and burnout. Our response to uncertainty can affect:

- **Our behaviour with the patient:** we may become more likely to carry out referrals or investigations, with the risk of unnecessary investigations or treatment and iatrogenic harm.

- **Our behaviour at work:** we may find ourselves over-working or becoming less efficient as we carry out excessive planning and preparation or repeating tasks as we double- and triple-check our work.

- **Our behaviour with others:** it may be hard to stop thinking about work or engage with family and friends due to excessive worry about possible problems. We may start to depend on repeated reassurance from others, which helps for a while but doesn't last.

We can understand some individual challenges to coping with uncertainty using a CBT framework (see figure below).

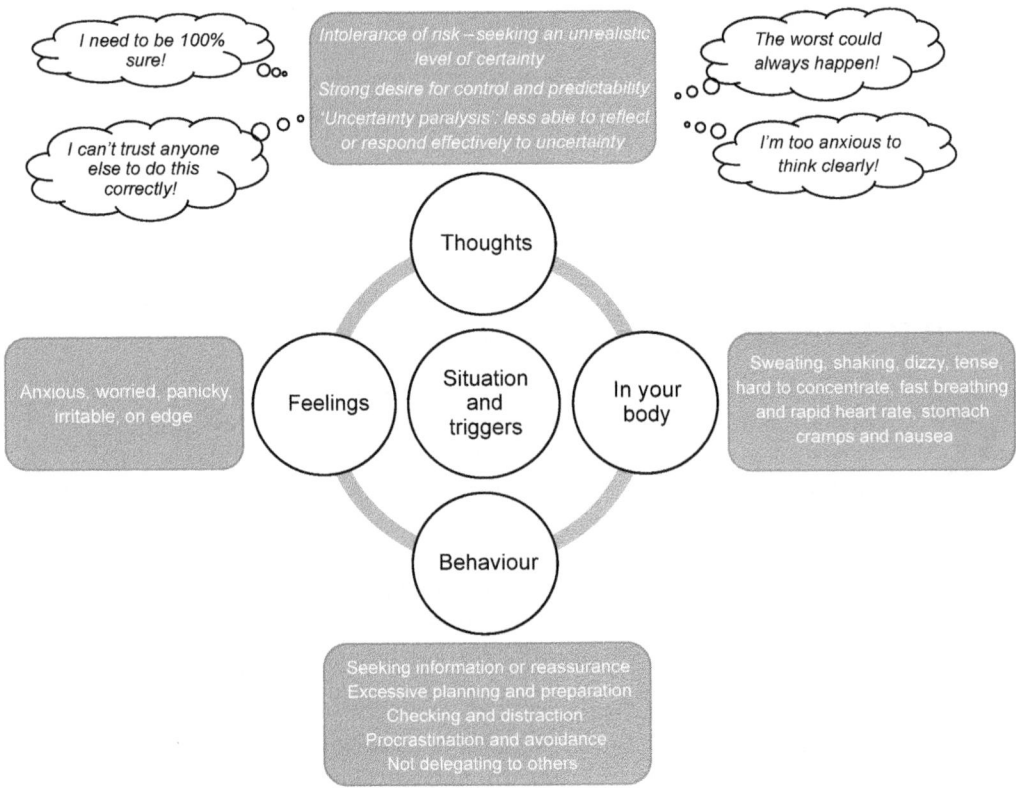

The ACCEPTS model of uncertainty

This model gives some helpful steps for health professionals to manage uncertainty:

- **A**cknowledge and **A**llow uncertainty
- **C**linical knowledge and judgement
- **C**ommunicate effectively
- **E**ngage in helpful behaviour
- **P**artnership and **P**ractice teams
- **T**est of **T**ime
- **S**elf-compassion

Acknowledge and Allow	The first step is to accept that uncertainty and complexity in general practice are inevitable and unavoidable, and we will be most effective at coping when we recognise and actively address, rather than trying to avoid these challenges. Good clinical care involves managing probabilities and learning to tolerate the discomfort and distress that uncertainty can trigger, rather than seeking an unrealistic or unhelpful level of certainty or avoiding decisions or action. See the ABLE method later in this chapter.
Clinical knowledge and judgement	Developing clinical knowledge, judgement and ultimately experience in making decisions about what to do, even if there is no precedent, helps with uncertainty. This means honing your ability to gather data and make balanced decisions that take into account a wide range of information, whilst ensuring that any knowledge gaps are minimised. This will aid your ability to generate hypotheses, consider a wide range of potential diagnoses and make informed decisions about investigations and management. It includes self-monitoring to recognise when you are feeling uncertain, and having flexibility to change and adapt to new information when needed.
Communicate effectively	Effective communication skills can improve your ability to gather information that may make a more accurate diagnosis. This is particularly important when coping with medical and social complexity and high levels of uncertainty. Communication also builds relationships and trust and may even reduce the risk of patient complaints. It can be helpful to develop communication skills for supporting patients who also find it difficult to tolerate uncertainty and may be experiencing anxiety about their health. Even small changes like slowing your pace of speech, making eye contact, checking understanding, and asking for feedback may help.

Engage in helpful behaviour	Engaging in helpful behaviour involves taking control over our own actions and making active choices about what is likely to be most helpful in the context of each unique situation. This includes making decisions about: • Balancing risk and harm: make balanced decisions about the use of tests and referrals based on clinical need rather than to 'reduce anxiety' • Cutting down unhelpful behaviours: remain thorough and build in checks and reminders but avoid excessive or repeated checking or reassurance-seeking, or deferring or avoiding decisions • Supporting your own wellbeing: find ways to care for yourself through healthy eating, regular exercise, social interaction and taking sufficient breaks at work.
Partnership and Practice teams	Developing partnerships with patients involves collaboration, and openly acknowledging and sharing risk and decision-making. Patients will generally accept uncertainty if it is skilfully handled, and if the clinician addresses the person's unique health beliefs and expectations. Practice teams involves working within a supportive environment which allows time to reflect and learn, and to engage in practice-based discussions about challenging cases and experiences of diagnostic uncertainty. This enables the uncertainty to be shared within the team and may facilitate more effective decision-making.
Test of time	The longitudinal nature of general practice means that time may be one of the most important strategies for managing uncertainty. This involves actively using safety-netting and follow-up to aid in making safe and effective diagnoses.
Self-compassion	Offer yourself kindness and compassion when facing complex and challenging situations at work, rather than judgement and self-criticism. It's important to be able to forgive yourself when things go wrong, or are outside your control, and to avoid perfectionist and unrealistic expectations of your own performance, or that of other people.

If you notice you are struggling with uncertainty, try using the following table to reflect on the ACCEPTS model:

Step of ACCEPTS model	Ask yourself:	What are your responses?
Acknowledge and Allow	• Am I seeking unrealistic levels of certainty in an uncertain situation? • Can I acknowledge, allow and cope with uncertainty and complexity rather than trying to eliminate it?	
Clinical knowledge and judgement	• What is my clinical judgement or intuition? What's most likely? • Is there anything serious that I need to consider or take into account? • Has any recent personal experience affected my perspective?	
Communicate effectively	• How could I use my communication skills to improve this situation? • What relationships are important (e.g. with patients, relatives, colleagues)?	
Engage in helpful behaviour	• What actions might help me cope with uncertainty (rather than seeking 100% certainty)? • Am I slipping into unhelpful checking, reassurance or compulsive actions? • What would be more helpful?	
Partnership (with colleagues and patients) and Practice teams	• How can I collaborate or seek partnership with the patient? • What support can I seek from colleagues? • How can I develop or strengthen my team?	
Test of time	• What is the expected course and progress? • How can I use safety-netting to support my decision? • What future signs might suggest complications or deterioration? • Have I told the patient how and when to seek help if concerned?	
Self-compassion	• What kind or supportive words and attitudes can I offer myself when coping with complexity and uncertainty? • What actions will help take care of myself, building my strength and resources to cope under challenging circumstances?	

ABLE to acknowledge and accept uncertainty

The **ABLE** model is a four-step approach to help you cope when struggling with any situation that involves uncertainty.

- **A**cknowledge and **A**llow: the first step is to notice when you are feeling a strong desire for certainty. Notice and give a name to the thoughts and feelings which arise, such as: "I'm thinking that I couldn't cope if things went wrong," or "I'm feeling anxious" or "I'm worrying about a particular risk or negative outcome." Allow the thoughts and feelings to be present without struggling to change them or to feel differently.

- **B**reathe: take a deep breath and exhale as slowly as possible. Repeat several times to create a *pause* and allow yourself time to *choose* what to do next.

- **L**abel your experiences and **L**et go of the need for certainty: try to observe if anxiety or discomfort around uncertainty has shown up. "I'm feeling tense, I'm worried that something might go wrong… I'm really wanting to be sure …". Remember, this thought or feeling will pass. You don't have to act on it, and trying to be 100% certain is not helpful or necessary and can get in the way of living your life.

- **E**xpand your attention and come back to doing something important right now. What were you doing before you started to worry? What action is likely to be most helpful in moving you towards a fulfilled, enjoyable life and is within your control? Use your five senses to connect to the activity fully: vision, hearing, touch, smell and taste.

9.8 GROWTH skills to cope with anxiety and uncertainty

There are many different skills and strategies that you can use to cope with anxiety, worry and uncertainty. It may take some time and experimentation to discover which approaches are most helpful for you personally.

Follow your inner Guide and be Ready for action

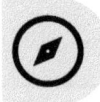

Remind yourself where your inner **Guide** is pointing. Are you neglecting any important values and needs because of anxiety? Are you avoiding important opportunities, or are actions such as repetitive checking getting in the way of living your life and being fully present in your relationships?

Following your **Guide** may involve facing challenges and uncertainty and taking difficult action, but it may be worth it in the pursuit of what matters. You could create some useful coping phrases and reminders, such as:

I don't want anxiety to stop me from doing what matters to me!

I want to stay focused and present when I'm with people I care about...

I want to reclaim my life from anxiety and have more choice and control...

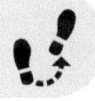

Take small steps to expand your opportunities and choice

Taking steps towards coping with anxiety and uncertainty may mean finding manageable ways to **approach** rather than avoid your fears. If anxiety has led to you limiting your life choices, then you can begin to choose actions that expand your options and possibilities.

Think back to the 'performance zones' that we met previously: the comfort zone, stretch zone, performance zone and the overload zone (see *Section 5.4*). Staying in the comfort zone may feel safer, but it also restricts your options and limits your life. If you spend all your time worrying about work problems or checking, what else are you missing out on? Perhaps there's a beautiful view, a chance to connect and enjoy time with friends or family, or simply time to have a little space to relax and find a sense of peacefulness.

We can choose actions that move us in the direction of our values, even if these involve facing anxiety and uncertainty. This is a bit like climbing a ladder – but you don't have to rush to the top – just take it one rung at a time! You can also enlist support to hold the ladder in place and encourage you until you feel steady. You might need to pause and take a break with each step, making sure your ladder doesn't wobble, and taking time to notice the lovely view from where you have reached!

You may also need to pause and make space so that you don't hit the overload zone, perhaps by reducing the challenge, seeking support, or giving yourself a little extra time to complete a bigger task.

Overload zone
Pause and make space **Engage coping strategies**
Performance zone
Stretch zone
Comfort zone

Values

Create your own anxiety ladder

You can use an anxiety ladder to plan small steps which gradually expand your life into the stretch and performance zones. Think of some ways that anxiety leads to Away actions that limit you or restrict your choices. There are some examples in the following table:

Away action	What's the impact of this on your life?	What are your most important values in this situation?	What small Towards step could you try as an alternative?
Avoiding challenges or situations that trigger anxiety			
Repeatedly asking for reassurance or engaging with doubt			
Over-checking, repeating actions, or excessive research of information			
Needing to distract yourself from anxiety in ways that are unhelpful in your wider life			
Procrastinating tasks, or putting off getting started on them because of anxiety			

EXERCISE: Moving up your anxiety ladder

Now choose one area that's important to your personal wellbeing. Create your own ladder below, which gradually increases the level of challenge as you move up through the zones. For each step, make a note of responses to the following questions:

- Why is this important to you to try?

- What will you do? When and where will you try it?

- What support can you seek out to help you make progress up the ladder?

- What skills can you use to help you successfully cope?

Remember at each step you can pause for a moment, make the challenge smaller, or repeat a step, before moving up to the next rung.

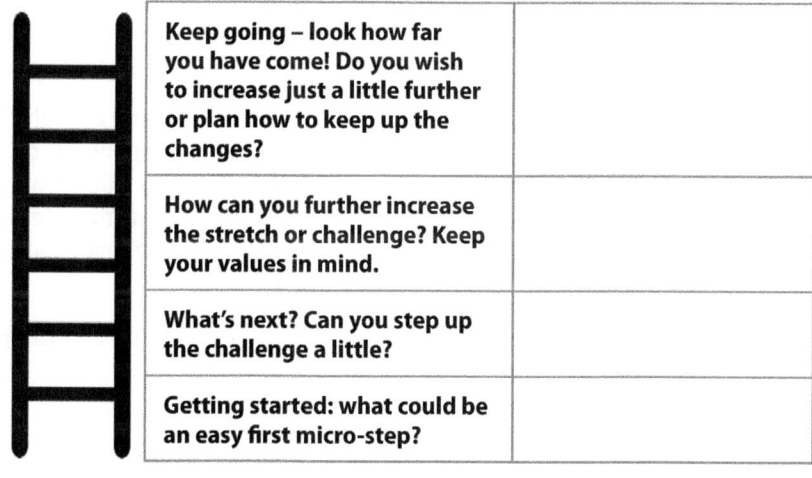

Keep going – look how far you have come! Do you wish to increase just a little further or plan how to keep up the changes?	
How can you further increase the stretch or challenge? Keep your values in mind.	
What's next? Can you step up the challenge a little?	
Getting started: what could be an easy first micro-step?	

Open and Observe anxiety

We can use **Open and Observe** skills (*Chapter 3*) to improve awareness of our personal responses, creating space to make more helpful decisions and choices when facing anxiety and uncertainty.

Surfing uncertainty

Could you try observing skills by 'surfing' the worry or uncertainty? This involves riding the wave and letting go of the struggle to find unrealistic levels of certainty. Be patient, kind and use self-compassion to help yourself accept that the world can be an uncertain place.

You can also bring your attention on doing things that matter, focusing on living a full and enjoyable life, rather than expending immense effort and energy in always wanting to be 'sure.'

Make Wise choices

Wise Mind can help you make helpful decisions about what to do and how to cope when you start to feel anxious. This involves choosing to listen to your inner coach and follow your inner **Guide**, rather than listening to the demands of the anxious mind visitors, who pop in uninvited.

The endless roundabout of worry….

Anxious thoughts often involve unanswerable 'what if…?' questions about the future. The incredible ability of our minds to think and reflect allows us to be creative, problem-solve and make complex diagnostic decisions. But this superpower also brings the capacity to imagine the worst possible outcomes and create ideas and stories about possible catastrophic future outcomes. We may also engage in questioning, doubting and seeking certainty by repeatedly looking for information and answers to things we are unsure about, which can become a never-ending cycle of worry.

Worry is a survival skill developed by humans, allowing us to think ahead and plan how to cope with possible danger before it happens. We can problem-solve, keep safe, and can prevent things from going wrong. But not all problems can be solved by thinking them through, especially events that are in the future. So, we may get stuck on a worry roundabout, endlessly thinking about the same *potential* problems, over and over again.

This is when worry becomes unhelpful and can take up a lot of time and energy.

Use a revolving door

You don't have to talk back, argue or try to force your anxious mind visitors to leave. Allow them to come in and then to wander back out again in their own time through a revolving door! Give them a nod and acknowledge them by name as they pass through: 'There's the Scaremonger', 'Hi, Checker…'

Sometimes an anxiety visitor might bring an important message – so you can press pause, make space to listen and reflect for a short time, and then allow them to leave a little later.

You could also invite your inner coach to come in through the door, take a seat and stay for a while, so you get a **Wise** perspective and support with making decisions based on all the different points of view.

Look at the big picture

Worry and anxiety often bring tunnel vision. You can get fixated on all the worrying parts of a situation and miss all the enjoyable and interesting parts. Or perhaps you are forgetting all your skills, strengths and abilities!

Next time you are thinking about a situation that is making you anxious, try asking yourself:

- **Is this helpful?** Is the way you are thinking helping you to be the person you want to be and to do the things you care about?

- **Can you take a helicopter view?** Imagine yourself rising above the situation, so that you can see ALL sides from a distance and the big picture. How does this change things?

- **Shift perspective** – how would others see this? Can you see it from a colleague or friend's point of view?

- **What skills do you have?** What knowledge or expertise can you draw on in this situation? Do you need to trust more in your capacity to cope?

- **Take the test of time** – how might you see the situation in a week, six months, or five years?

Then bring your focus back to NOW. Don't try to stop or control your thoughts. Just put them on the 'back burner' whilst bringing your attention to an important task in the present moment.

Use a worry decision tree

Using a worry decision tree (see figure below) involves deciding whether a worry is something that you have some control over, and you can take some action on, or whether it's just something that *might* happen, or that you cannot control.

If you can do something about the worry, you can use problem-solving to think about what action to take, and then make a plan to carry out this action at a specific time. However, it's also important not to spend excessive amounts of time thinking about problem-solving – this may be another form of worry.

If you can't do anything about the problem right away, or the worry is about something that you can't control, you can shift your focus, using techniques such as ABLE to recognise the worry or uncertainty and then move on with your day.

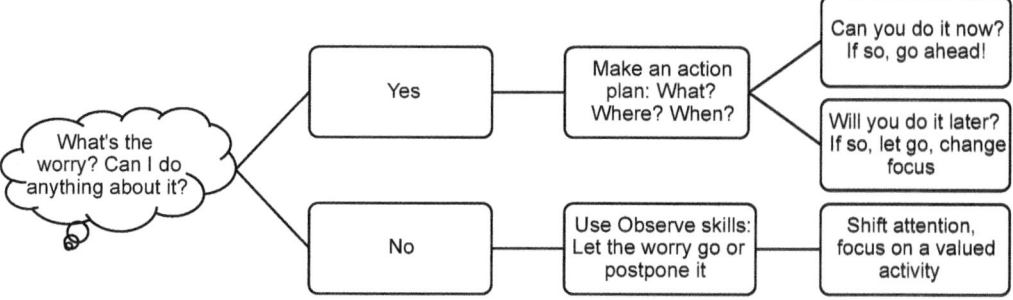

Plan thinking time

Thinking time involves choosing a regular convenient time to think about your worries and concerns. This gives your anxious mind opportunity to be heard – sometimes it may have something important to contribute! But it's also important not to spend your whole day going repeatedly round the worry roundabout.

If worries pop into your mind at other times, you can put them 'on hold' until your planned thinking time, using the following steps:

Step 1: Plan your thinking time: choose a slot of 15–30 minutes each day, ideally at the same time and in the same place, and preferably not just before bedtime.

Step 2: Put the worry 'on hold': if a worry pops into your mind at another time of day, tell yourself: *It's OK to have this worry, but I will deal with it later, during thinking time.*

If you are concerned about forgetting a worry, you can make a brief note in a journal or on your phone. After writing it down, close the book again until thinking time.

Step 3: Focus on what's important: after noting down your worry, bring your attention back onto the present moment, and concentrate on whatever activity you are carrying out.

Don't be concerned if the same thought soon pops back up again. It is common to have repeated worry thoughts. Just repeat the process: accept the thought, make a note, and put it on hold for later.

Step 4: Allow your thinking time: now it's time to think about these problems as much as you like! Look through your list of worries or problems and cross anything off the list that's no longer a concern. Use problem-solving to help overcome any practical problems.

Continue thinking and problem-solving for no more than 15–30 minutes. You might need to set a timer to remind you when to stop! Then, move on to another activity that is likely to take your mind away from your worries and lift your mood, such as exercise, listening to music or calling a friend.

Plan how to cope

Worry often involves recurrent 'what if…?' thoughts about potential problems and catastrophes. But managing worry shouldn't just involve reassuring yourself the worst won't happen. It's often more helpful to focus on developing your self-belief and confidence that you could cope if things did go wrong, shifting focus from 'what if…?' to 'then what…?' Having a 'Plan B' can also help settle anxiety.

Think of a recurrent worry or a 'what if…?' thought, such as: "What if I'm really busy and I run really late?", "What if a patient makes a complaint?" or "What if I make a prescribing error because I'm rushing?".

Now, ask yourself: "Then what would I do?" "If things really did go wrong, how might I cope?" Use the following table to help guide your answer:

What skills or experience do you have that might help you cope with the problem if it arose?	
What help, advice or support could you obtain from other people?	
What practical steps could you take that would make a start in coping or dealing with the situation?	
Is it helpful to focus on 'what if…?' thoughts and worries? What's the impact of getting stuck on the worry roundabout?	
What does your inner coach say? What's a compassionate and wise perspective on the problem?	
Right now, what's the most helpful thing you could do next?	

Paola uses this approach to reflect on some of her worries:

"I do have a lot of 'what if…?' worry thoughts! I usually try to reassure myself, but I can see that this often doesn't last long, and I just end up worrying again. One of my main worries is that I might mis-read a result or not action something important in a letter."

What skills or experience do you have that might help you cope with the problem if it arose?	I don't often miss things – I'm usually very careful. But if I did make a mistake, I could try to draw on my inner coach and be kind to myself. I would feel really bad about it, because I care about doing a good job for my patients.
What help, advice or support could you obtain from other people?	If I did miss something, I could ask my colleagues for support. We could discuss it at a significant event meeting and look for what we could learn as a team. Someone else in the team might pick up the problem before it becomes a major issue.

What practical steps could you take that would make a start in coping or dealing with the situation?	If I did miss something, I would contact the patient and take action to ensure that any harm was minimised.
Is it helpful to focus on 'what if...?' thoughts and worries? What's the impact of getting stuck on the worry roundabout?	It definitely doesn't help me to keep thinking about this – spending too much time worrying about making a mistake probably makes me more likely to miss something because it's hard to concentrate!
What does your inner coach say? What's a compassionate and wise perspective on the problem?	My inner coach would say that it's important not to allow worry about a mistake to become overpowering or influence my work too greatly. I need to be kind and understanding about how hard it is to get everything right all the time. All I can do is my best.
Right now, what's the most helpful thing you could do next?	When I'm stuck in worrying about making a mistake, it's important to bring my attention back to working effectively and focus on the patient in front of me.

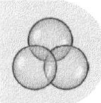

Thrive and Balance the threat system

Keeping your stress bucket at a reasonable level will prevent the build-up of anxiety and emotional snapping. A really important strategy for managing anxiety and uncertainty is to step out of the threat system, creating more balance and stability by engaging your drive system, and engaging your calm and connect systems using self-compassion. We talk about this in more detail in *Chapter 5*.

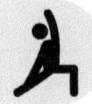

Healthy Life Habits

Creating and maintaining healthy routines can help to manage physical and emotional tension and help you cope better with feelings of anxiety and improve your overall wellbeing. Important areas may include developing healthy habits around physical activity, sleep, alcohol, caffeine and your use of technology and social media. Turn back to *Chapter 6* and think about establishing some **Healthy Life Habits** to create a platform of wellbeing for your body and mind.

Chapter summary: Anxiety and uncertainty

- Managing uncertainty is an inherent part of the challenge and emotional demands that arise when working in primary care.

- Anxiety is a normal response when you perceive a threat, but can become a problem if it starts to restrict or interfere with how you live your daily life.

- GROWTH skills for managing anxiety include:
  - following your inner **Guide** without allowing anxiety or fear of uncertainty to pull you away from what matters most
  - taking small steps towards important activities that you may be avoiding or putting off due to anxiety
  - using **Open and Observe** to notice when your anxious mind has shown up, creating space to step back and allowing worry thoughts to wander back out through a revolving door
  - seeking a wider perspective, recognising that fears are not facts, 'surfing' worry and making Wise choices that are helpful for you personally
  - maintaining your general wellbeing and reducing baseline stress levels to Thrive and engage with **Healthy Life Habits**.

Final thoughts

What are the most important messages for you from this chapter?

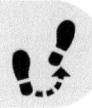

Take an action step

What are your next steps? What actions will you take as a result of reading this chapter?

Are there any regular actions or patterns of behaviour that you might try to practise or develop to cope more effectively with anxiety or uncertainty?

10 Connecting and communicating

- Do you feel isolated or in need of more connection to colleagues, friends or family?

- Are you a people person who thrives on social interaction or do you need time and space alone to reflect and recharge?

- Are you able to empathise with others yet assert your own needs, and confidently resolve conflicts or have 'difficult' conversations?

- Could strengthening relationships improve your wellbeing and happiness? Keep reading…

10.1 The importance of connection

Effective relationships, both one-to-one and within a team, are essential to our roles as health professionals. Strong connections with colleagues, friends and family can provide a sense of belonging, offer a support network when life is tough, and be a source of happiness, contentment and fun.

Relationships also play an important role in wellbeing. Feelings of connection arise from the quality of our relationships and our personality traits, rather than the number of friends or colleagues we have. You can feel happy alone, enjoying the peace of your own company, and you can also feel isolated or lonely, even when surrounded by people in a busy surgery, or within your own family.

The nature of healthcare or management roles can engender a sense of responsibility and also loneliness. Perhaps you are experiencing relationship difficulties at work, or in your personal life, or you might be coping with a change in circumstances such as moving to a new area, promotion, or working with a new team. These situations can all result in busy clinicians experiencing feelings of disconnection or isolation.

When relationships are strained at work, we may start to feel anxious, low and irritable. We might react by lashing out at others, avoiding social situations, or turning to negative coping strategies such as alcohol, drugs, technology or comfort eating.

In this chapter we will look at:

- how personality traits such as extraversion and introversion can influence how we interact with others and the types of relationship we enjoy or find supportive
- ways to strengthen existing important relationships and expand our relationship circles to reduce feelings of isolation
- strategies to overcome social and performance-related anxiety
- communication skills for resolving conflict and having difficult conversations

Marija, GP: *"I'm originally from Croatia and I moved to the UK with my husband 10 years ago. Most of our family support is at home in Croatia. We have moved around for work, so it's been hard to make and keep friendships. Also, I'm not very outgoing, and I prefer solitary activities to unwind from work. Recently, I've been feeling more and more disconnected, and it is now affecting my mood and motivation. I've been working at my current practice for a few years now. I am always polite and friendly, but I keep myself at a distance as I'm never sure what to say if it is not about work or how the surgery is running. I feel quite isolated, and I don't feel I have much in common with the other GPs in the practice."*

What possible signs of disconnection or isolation can you notice in the example?

Can you recognise any similar signs in yourself? Note them here:

10.2 Personality traits and relationships

Our personality traits can influence how we form relationships and connect with others. Understanding your own tendencies, and those of the people around you, may help to build stronger relationships, maximise your personal strengths, and cope more effectively with any vulnerabilities or potential difficulties.

Extrovert personalities

Extroverts are typically outgoing, sociable individuals. They are strong communicators who find it easy to form relationships with a wide range of people. Extroverts are usually confident in the spotlight and enjoy speaking publicly. They are often charismatic, with strong leadership qualities, and a high level of enthusiasm and energy which can be infectious and motivating for others. They are 'big picture' thinkers who work well in groups and prefer to understand and solve problems through collaborative discussion. Extroverts are often proactive people who like getting involved in many different activities and are good at making things happen.

Introvert personalities

Introverts are typically more quiet, reflective, analytical and reserved individuals, who prefer to think before taking action. They feel comfortable spending time alone and energise through peaceful or solitary activities. They are self-aware, insightful and empathetic and are good listeners, who value other people's perspectives but often prefer one-to-one interactions or smaller groups. They are usually balanced, fair and thoughtful leaders, who lead through mentorship and encouragement. People with introvert traits can be precise and detail-oriented, and their ability to focus makes them highly effective at managing projects. They are often self-motivated, able to take the lead and make decisions and offer practical solutions. Introverts are often composed and able to manage their emotions well, enabling them to cope with problems and difficulties.

Understanding your personal traits

Here are some examples of personality traits that reflect extrovert and introvert characteristics. Do you recognise any of these? How do they affect you, your wellbeing and how you relate to others?

Example of personality trait	Possible challenges with this trait	Do you recognise this?
You have high levels of enthusiasm and are keen to get moving with projects and ideas.	You may sometimes find it hard to listen to others or take on board what they are saying.	
You are energetic and motivated, and willing to take on multiple projects.	It can be hard to meet deadlines and you may not allow sufficient time for thinking and planning. You may take on too many tasks and become overwhelmed.	
You are a confident speaker who is articulate and thrives in the spotlight.	Appearing over-confident or stealing the limelight can create resentment in others, who may not feel valued or acknowledged.	

You are expressive and charismatic, wearing your 'heart on your sleeve'. You motivate others with your infectious enthusiasm and positive emotions.	At times it may be difficult (for you and others) to cope with your extreme emotional swings from enthusiasm to despondency and overwhelm.	
You enjoy being stimulated through interaction with others, or by an exciting task or environment.	You can become bored and lose interest if working in isolation, and find it hard to complete repetitive, mundane tasks.	
You are able to take decisive and immediate action when needed.	You may be impulsive, which can cause problems with complex projects that need detailed planning.	
You prefer to focus on one project at a time in a detailed and thorough way.	You may find it stressful or become overwhelmed and irritable if you have multiple challenges to cope with simultaneously.	
You are autonomous and self-motivated. You work well in a quiet environment and when there's a clear plan for when and how to interact with others.	You may find external stimuli distracting and get frustrated with frequent interruptions when focused on a task. You may struggle with giving ad hoc advice or informal collaboration.	
You are a dependable and reliable member of the team who may be quiet or introspective until you feel comfortable and know others better.	You might sometimes be perceived as aloof or distant and find it hard to build relationships quickly.	
You are thoughtful and reflective and think things through in detail. You have a strong sense of the best way to approach a project.	You might become over-focused on the details or on your own thoughts and forget to check that your ideas fit the reality or needs of others. You need time to process feedback from others and to be persuaded to shift your opinion.	
You enjoy interactions one-to-one or in small groups and you are a good listener who remembers details about other people.	You may find working in groups, attending meetings, public speaking and social events tiring, stressful or a source of anxiety. You may be unassertive or drowned out by more dominant personalities.	
You are thorough and prefer to avoid unnecessary risks. You research every angle and potential obstacle thoroughly before making decisions.	You may become overly risk-averse and lack flexibility when facing changing circumstances. You may be unwilling to make rapid decisions, even if these are necessary, causing frustration for others.	

Here are some strategies and tips for ways to balance both extrovert and introvert personality traits.

Balancing extrovert traits

- **Boost your energy with social interaction:** include enough time to interact during your week. If you often work alone, ensure you leave your room and have a chat at lunchtime, or plan a catch-up with a group of friends after work. Can you do some work tasks in a shared space, so you are able to liaise with other members of the practice team for part of the day?

- **Pause and check in:** to combat any tendency to jump in before thinking, try taking a moment to pause and check in with yourself. Take a slow exhale or use your five senses to engage body and mind, noticing any urges to take impulsive action.

- **Encourage others to contribute:** ensure your enthusiasm is not making you over-dominant. Listen carefully to others and encourage quieter or less confident individuals to contribute. Give others time to reflect on your questions by circulating discussion points in advance, rather than putting someone on the spot.

- **Plan your time:** extroverts seek frequent stimulation and avoid alone time, so often have packed and exhausting schedules. Take a look at the section on 'hurry habits' in *Chapter 6*. Keep your targets reasonable and realistic, and schedule in a little time to give yourself a break from others and some time and space to recharge.

Balancing introvert traits

- **Practise acting 'as if' you are a little more extrovert:** make an effort to make eye contact, smile, speak clearly and express your opinion in small group situations to develop your public speaking skills in less threatening situations. Behave 'as if' you feel a little more confident or are just a little more extrovert.

- **Plan for challenging situations:** ask to see the agenda before a difficult meeting, so you have time to prepare your thoughts and what you might say, including a plan for how you might overcome possible problems or difficulties. Then make time and space to recharge afterwards.

- **Use active listening:** your natural strength is listening, so use your curiosity to join in and ask questions that show genuine interest in what others are saying.

- **Develop important relationships:** pick one or two people that you would like to know better and focus on enhancing these relationships. Be brave and take small steps towards strengthening these connections.

- **Seek support when under pressure:** your tendency to internalise stresses and difficulties means that you may be less likely to turn to others for support, which can make you isolated. Remember to actively seek support and share your feelings with others to help you through difficult times.

10.3 Relationship circles

We have many different types of relationships in our lives, which vary in how close you feel and how well you know the other person. These include:

- **Close family:** your closest relationships are usually at home, including your partner, children and pets.

- **Supporters:** these are close friends and colleagues that you can trust and confide in and who provide support in difficult times.

- **Wider friends and colleagues:** these are people who you see regularly at work or in other areas of life, but who you do not have a close relationship with.

- **Acquaintances:** people that you don't know well or you just know by sight.

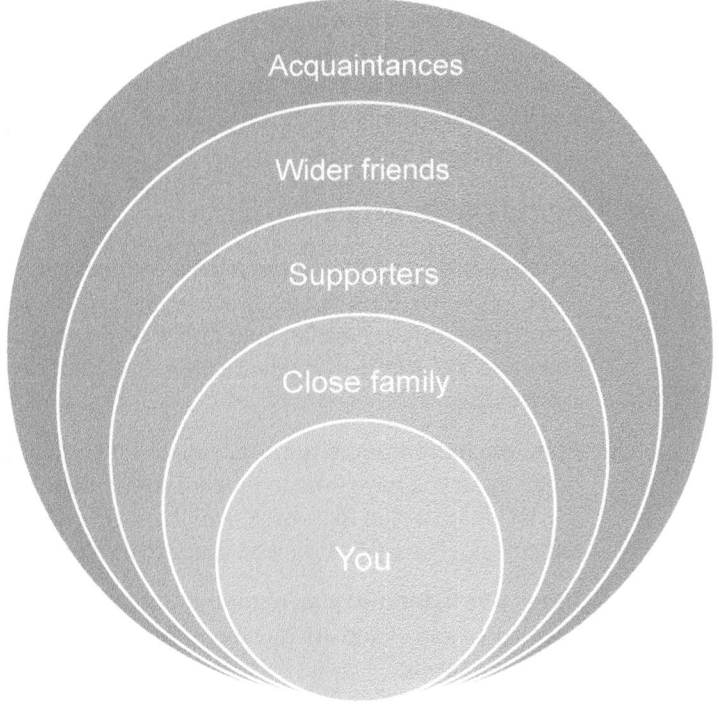

10.4 Strengthening important relationships

Our inner **Guide** often points towards relationships as being central to our sense of meaning, purpose and wellbeing. Would you benefit from taking time to strengthen your important and close relationships? Here are some tips:

Tips for improving close relationships	How might this help? What could you try?
Find something you both enjoy Could you plan to watch a movie, play a board game, go for a walk or cook a meal together?	
Show you are interested Ask questions and be genuinely curious about what the person is saying. Try just being a supportive listening ear – don't feel responsible for solving the problem or jump in with your own story or opinion.	
Make time and minimise distractions What places or situations make it easier to relax and give your full attention? Chatting whilst driving in the car or walking next to someone may ease the pressure. Put your phone in your pocket and resist the temptation to check it during the conversation.	
Laughter is the best medicine Humour is a great way to connect. This could be anything from sharing a joke, playing a game, going to a comedy night or watching a TV programme together.	
Reconnect with an old friend Have you lost contact with someone who has moved away or stopped doing a shared activity? Can you find creative new ways to grow your relationship in changing circumstances?	
Add your own ideas: how else could you deepen your connection to close friends and family?	

10.5 Expanding relationship circles

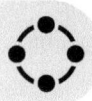

There may also be times in life that you would benefit from expanding your friendship circles. This may take time, perseverance and some effort. But the rewards that come from increasing your close and trusted connections may be worth working at.

There are many different ways to widen your relationship circles. Try not to put yourself under pressure to develop relationships. Focus on enjoying being around people with shared interests and allowing feelings of connection to build slowly and naturally. Think about what is important to you and what different interests you have that might be shared with others. Just a few examples include:

Physical activity: join a walking, running or cycling group, a tennis or golf club, or a football or netball team	**Volunteer your time:** support a local organisation or charity such as Scouts or Guides, a homeless charity, or get involved with the PTA or become a governor at a local school
Expand your casual acquaintances: ask a neighbour to go for a dog walk or to have a coffee	**Creativity and practical activities:** get involved in groups or classes, e.g. art, pottery, craft, gardening, DIY or carpentry
Local community: join a local book group, the Women's Institute, a residents' committee, or a pub quiz team; if there's nothing suitable, consider starting your own group	**Spiritual and religious activities:** involve yourself in activities relating to your faith, or join a meditation group
Education and learning: sign up for a diploma, or something unrelated to work, and find others with a shared interest	**Music and performance:** get involved with a local choir or orchestra or tread the boards or help backstage with a drama production

PAUSE AND REFLECT: Strengthening connections

- Are you experiencing disconnection or isolation?
- Do any of the ideas above seem relevant or useful? What else might help?
- What might be your first steps?

Marija, GP: *"I am quite an introvert and I do find it hard to build relationships with others, although I'm a great friend once you get to know me! I'm going to make an effort at work to 'behave as if' I feel just a little more confident. I've picked out a couple of other quiet people in the practice who seem friendly, and I will make an effort to say hello when I get to work or at lunchtime. There are some practice social events that I've never gone along to. I was thinking of asking one of the more friendly receptionists whether she is going, and perhaps I might go too. I'll pick something that doesn't seem too stressful to get started, such as going to a local music concert that means I won't have to chat so much. I'm also wondering about signing up to a sewing course as I've always wanted to learn and we will be quite busy during the classes, so I won't have to worry so much about what to say."*

10.6 Social and performance stress

Many situations can trigger performance stress. You might feel anxious in large groups, speaking up at a meeting, performing a practical procedure, parking your car in front of others, or competing in a sport. These situations can trigger fears about looking foolish and not living up to the expectations of ourselves or others. Performance stress can arise in people who are not usually anxious, and in people who have a high standard or ability in the activity they are participating in.

George, GP Registrar: *"I carried out an audit at my practice and my Trainer was really positive about it. She encouraged me to share the results with the practice at a lunchtime meeting.*
I started feeling really nervous. I couldn't stop thinking that I would mess it up or make a fool of myself. They are a group of very experienced GPs and nurses! What if they disagreed with my conclusions or discovered that I'd made a mistake in my slides? Once as a student, I got really nervous when giving a talk and I kept tripping over my words. It would be very embarrassing if that happened again. I was also really worried about what questions they might ask, so I started to over-prepare to a ridiculous level and it took up all my free time."

10.7 What gets in the way?

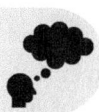

Many different fears and worries might pop up when we are experiencing social or performance-related stress and anxiety. Some examples include:

Connection and performance-blocking thoughts and fears	Do you recognise this?
Catastrophic worries about all the things that might go wrong	
Ignoring your past achievements and times that things have gone well	
Imagining other people disagreeing, laughing or judging you negatively	
Thoughts about being less interesting or competent than peers	
Lacking confidence or underestimating your ability to cope with the challenges of the situation	
Memories or images of yourself looking foolish or awkward, or stumbling over your words	
Worrying about being in the spotlight with everyone staring at you	
Extreme high standards and perfectionist expectations about how you should perform	

PAUSE AND REFLECT: The impact of negative thoughts or fears

What's the impact of these thoughts? How do they alter your behaviour in social or performance situations?

Coping with negative thoughts and feelings

Remember, these thoughts are simply opinions and guesses about what might happen, not absolute facts. It's not necessary to believe or 'buy into' the thoughts if they are unhelpful or getting in the way of living or working. Giving a lot of attention to negative thoughts can increase your anxiety and you may get stuck in a negative spiral where you avoid interactions or keep others at a distance.

Look back at some of the ways you learnt to deal with unhelpful thinking in previous chapters. Can you step back and see things from the perspective of your

Wise Mind or Wise inner coach? How would you behave differently if you took this perspective? Is your threat system over-reacting? Can you show yourself some compassion and care as you prepare? Think back to *Section 5.6* on ways to **Thrive and Balance**.

Where is your attention?

When feeling anxious in a social or performance situation, it's common to turn your attention inwards. You put your performance under the spotlight to ensure that you don't do or say anything foolish or incorrect, and focus on:

- Catastrophic thoughts and negative stories about how things might go wrong

- Being hyper-aware of your body and any physical sensations of anxiety, such as a racing heart, sweaty palms or how much you are blushing

- Worrying about how you are coming across and repeatedly planning and rehearsing what to say next

- Jumping to negative conclusions when you notice someone yawn or glance at their watch, assuming it means they are bored or judging you negatively.

Excessive self-focus makes it harder to listen to or interact with the people around you. You're also more likely to notice any subtle symptoms of anxiety in your body, which makes you feel worse as you jump to conclusions about how anxious you appear to others. And placing yourself under excessive pressure can increase feelings of anxiety and may even worsen your performance.

Training your attention

One of the best ways of overcoming performance-related stress is to shift your focus away from yourself and how you are being perceived and connect with your audience, the environment, the task or the people around you. Use your skills in being **Open and Observing** the present moment to bring your awareness to whatever you are doing.

Next time you notice that your attention has wandered away from a conversation try coming back to the topic at hand, listening closely to what the other person is saying. You can use your senses to ground yourself in the present moment, looking at the colours in the room, noticing any sounds around you, becoming aware of the pressure of your feet on the ground, or taking a slow sip of your drink. There are many open and observe exercises to build this skill in *Chapter 3*.

You can also use this to steady yourself during a performance situation, drawing your attention back from thoughts about looking foolish or messing up your words, and bringing your focus back to the present moment. You can draw on your **Wise Mind** to offer support, guidance and compassion, rather than getting caught up in perfectionist rules about how you 'should' perform.

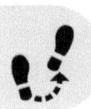

Action steps for creating connection

To develop relationships, we need to be present and give out signals that we are friendly and willing to connect. Here are some of our tips for increasing connection with those around you.

Schedule time for connection: arriving a little early to work or to a group activity will give you the chance to chat informally to others and get to know people.

Notice who is around you: try widening your focus of attention to include other people. Making just brief eye contact and a smile can be important steps for making connections.

Be open to opportunities: think of your body language as you enter a room. Smile and say hello to someone or sit next to someone to eat your lunch and ask how their day is going. Remember to pay attention to their answer, rather than focusing on thinking about what to say next!

Expand your circles of support: try not to place too many expectations or demands on any one relationship. Aim to have a range of people who you can connect with for your varied interests and needs, and a smaller number of people with which you feel comfortable to share personal feelings or experiences.

Act with confidence: if you are feeling nervous about talking to someone or giving a presentation, remember that it's possible to act with confidence even when negative thoughts and feelings, such as doubts and uncertainty, show up. Plan coping strategies for dealing with potential problems, such as making a joke if there are IT problems, and then continue with your talk.

Manage your expectations: is it realistic to think that your presentation must be perfect, or that you should never make a mistake in front of others? Choose to listen to your supportive inner coach rather than your critic. Can you offer understanding and acceptance rather than judgement and blame, as you find ways to cope in difficult circumstances?

George, GP Registrar: "*I decided that I would just do my best with the presentation and not put myself under pressure to do it perfectly. My Trainer was there to offer support and said she would be happy to step in for any difficult questions. I practised getting my slides onto the computer the day before, and it was a good thing as there were some problems in getting connected. This made it a lot smoother on the day.*
Just before the presentation, I started feeling very nervous and shaky. All the worry thoughts came rushing back. I took a slow breath and used my five senses while having a couple of sips of cold water to bring myself back to the present moment. Then I tried to bring my full attention to the topic at hand – I focused

> *on talking steadily and getting my message across clearly. It wasn't perfect but I managed to get through without too many slips. Afterwards, the senior partner congratulated me and said I had done a good job – I was really pleased!"*

10.8 Communication and managing conflict

Effective communication is essential for building relationships, and helps us to manage conflict or disagreement, enabling us to work with others and within teams. Most clinicians are excellent communicators, both professionally and in social situations. However, even with these skills and experience, communicating with others is not always straightforward. Working in primary care is busy and demanding and involves interacting with a wide range of people with differing personalities, beliefs and opinions. This is compounded by the many pressures of work, which can mean that conflict and misunderstandings are sometimes inevitable with both colleagues and patients. This can lead to frustration, stress and disconnection.

Assertiveness

Assertiveness involves using clear and honest communication which expresses your own feelings, needs and opinions, whilst recognising those of other people. It's not about being forceful, rude or aggressive, or making other people do what you want. These kinds of behaviour may mean that the person gets their own way, but can negatively affect relationships with others, who may feel hurt or disrespected.

At times we may lack assertiveness. Giving in, or not expressing your views may seem easier than being honest or facing a potential confrontation. But being unable to contribute can leave you feeling frustrated and powerless, as you lose the chance to get recognition and positive feedback for your ideas and expertise.

Confident compassionate communication

Confident compassionate communication is an alternative to giving in or being overly dominant. It can help you to manage conflict and difficult conversations, and to express your needs to others. It involves being able to:

- Express your ideas, opinions, and feelings openly, directly and honestly

- Stand up for your own rights while respecting those of others

- Take responsibility for yourself and your actions without judging or blaming other people

- Take other people's perspectives and needs into account

- Find ways to connect, cooperate and compromise when dealing with disagreements or conflict.

Confident compassionate communication involves four steps, which involve getting **NEAR** to others:

- **N**otice and describe the situation without judgement
- **E**motions: recognise and express how you are feeling
- **A**sk yourself what matters most (to you and the other person)
- **R**easonable request – what might help meet your/their needs?

Notice and describe the situation

Everyday communication is filled with interpretations and opinions, which often involves analysing, judging or criticising other people. But expressing things in this way can be unhelpful during a conflict or disagreement.

Instead, we can *notice* and *describe* the situation without judgement. This involves focusing on the objective, observable facts. What happened? What could be seen or heard?

PAUSE AND REFLECT: Dropping judgemental language

Look at these different ways of talking about a problem. For the first few examples, we have included some judgements and suggested an alternative that involves describing and observing. Can you complete the final examples? Feel free to adapt the situation to make it more relevant to your own life and experiences.

Interpretations, blaming or criticising	Non-judgemental describing
It was a terrible morning, and my day was ruined by the appalling traffic!	There was a lot of traffic this morning which made me late for an important appointment
You were so snappy and rude when you got home from work	I noticed that you were brusque when I asked how your day was
I'm so useless in meetings, I never get my point across	I didn't speak up when my manager asked what we wanted to do about the problem
You are so irritating and annoying…	
He is so lazy…	

The problem is that you're too selfish	
She is so irresponsible!	

The aim is to express yourself clearly and honestly without judgements or blame. This can be very challenging! It helps to use our **Open and Observe** skills to recognise any habitual ways of thinking or talking, and step back to more neutral and descriptive language.

Pitfalls	Avoid saying...	What could you say instead?
Making judgements	*You should...* *You never...* *You are...*	*I noticed that...* *I'm hoping for...* *I'm wondering if...*
Blaming (yourself or others)	*You shouldn't be so careless!* *It's your (my) fault!*	*I feel disappointed because...* *I'm wishing that...*
Advising, correcting or explaining	*Your problem is that...* *What you should do is...*	*This seems difficult...* *I'm worried that this happened...*
Storytelling and 'one-upping'	*You think that's bad!* *Let me tell you about the time that I...*	*I'm remembering some similar experiences, but I'd like to hear your thoughts first...*
Making demands	*I need you to...* *You have to...* *I want...*	*What's important to me is...* *I'm hoping for...*
Name-calling and criticism	*You're such an idiot!* *You're so incompetent!*	*I can see that something has gone wrong...* *It looks like an important step was missed...*

Emotions: recognise and express how you are feeling

Recognising your emotions may help you to understand what's important and what might improve a difficult situation. This can be tricky, especially when the feelings are strong or arise quickly.

Ask yourself:

- How do I feel about this? What emotions can I notice?

- What's driving this? What's behind my reaction?

Try to name your feelings and express them using "I" statements, saying: *"I'm feeling frustrated… hurt… excited… hopeful…".* And if talking about emotions is uncomfortable, you can leave out the word 'feeling' by saying, *"I'm disappointed by this situation…"* or *"I'm frustrated…".*

It can help to build your vocabulary of feelings to develop your self-understanding and knowledge. Some examples of feelings when our needs are being met include:

Comfortable Satisfied, at ease, rested	**Grateful** Appreciative, thankful	**Friendly** Amiable, receptive, open
Energised Refreshed, alert, determined, powerful	**Playful** Adventurous, inspired, stimulated, excited, eager	**Loving** Connected, warm, affectionate, tender
Interested Curious, excited, enthusiastic, proud	**Peaceful** Calm, content, relaxed, safe	**Happy** Glad, joyful, hopeful, cheerful, delighted

Common feelings when our needs are NOT being met include:

Angry Irritable, frustrated, annoyed, furious, fed up	**Scared** Anxious, worried, insecure, fearful, panicky, terrified	**Sad** Unhappy, lonely, gloomy, miserable
Frozen Shocked, stuck, shut off, numb	**Uncertain** Confused, hesitant, unsure	**Embarrassed** Envious, jealous, ashamed
Disappointed Bitter, upset, hurt	**Uninterested** Tired, fed up, bored	**Uncomfortable** Uneasy, in pain

Ask yourself what matters most

Think about why the situation is important to you and what matters to the other person. Conflicts often arise when people have different opinions about what would be the best strategy to deal with a particular problem. Instead, it's often helpful to pause and think about our needs and values before discussing what action to take. This encourages connection and builds relationships, and also creates space to be creative and brainstorm different ways of dealing with things, rather than insisting that there is only one way to solve a complex problem.

Ask yourself:

- What personal values and needs are relevant to this situation?

- Why is this situation important to you?

- What could matter to the other person? Can you make a guess about their needs and values? How are these different or similar to yours?

We talked in more detail about values and needs in *Chapter 1*. Here's a reminder of some common needs which may be important in relationships:

- **Acceptance**: empathy, love, respect, support, approval

- **Acknowledgement:** to matter, to be valued, appreciated, heard, seen, respected, recognised

- **Autonomy:** choice, independence, freedom, power, responsibility, space, consent

- **Belonging:** communication, community, cooperation, inclusion, participation, sharing

- **Connection:** affection, appreciation, closeness, warmth, care, partnership

- **Enjoyment:** fun, play, laughter, excitement, celebration, humour

- **Meaning and purpose:** contribution, effectiveness, fulfilment, achievement, using skills, creativity

- **Safety and security:** financial and physical

- **Sense of self:** authenticity, integrity, self-acceptance and self-compassion, dignity, mourning

- **Trust:** honesty, equality, fairness, certainty, loyalty

- **Understanding:** awareness, clarity, learning, discovery, growth, stimulation, exploration.

Reasonable request

The final step involves thinking about what to do next and involves making a reasonable request to yourself or the other person. A reasonable request is not a demand. This means that the other person has the choice to say 'no' without being threatened with any negative consequences. It also involves asking for something that the other person has the power to achieve. Asking a colleague for world peace or a loan of £1 million might be outside most people's control!

When planning a reasonable request, be creative and keep everyone's needs and values in mind. Try to find some common ground and think about things you agree on.

Ask yourself:

- What solutions might find a balance or a compromise, or are mutually acceptable or agreeable?
- How can you express the request in a way that's respectful and likely to be received well?

Some examples of reasonable requests include:

- Could you help me understand and explain why you made that decision?
- Can you tell me how you feel about what happened and what you would like me to do differently next time?
- Could you give me some time to think about your request?
- Can you tell me what you heard me say?

Confident compassionate communication in action

Helena, Practice Nurse: *"I've been off work for a few weeks after an operation. I'm due back to work next week but I don't feel completely well and I'm worried that if I come back too soon it will have a negative effect on my recovery. I've got a meeting with the practice manager next week and I'm feeling really anxious about it. He is a really effective manager and a strong character, used to getting on with things, and he doesn't always give me time to get my point across. He's expecting that I will be ready to come back straight away, and I know how short-staffed they are at the moment. I'm worried that he will think I'm shirking my duties or that I don't care about my job. I don't know how to tell him that I'm not ready in a way that won't get him frustrated and will show that I am committed to my work."*

Plan and prepare	Choose the best time and place for a conversation, which doesn't ambush or surprise the person. Think in advance what you would like to achieve and what you can say.	I will send the practice manager an email to confirm I'm coming for the meeting next week and warn him that I'm not as well as I'd like, and I would like to talk about the next steps for my return to work. I'll spend some time practising what I might say before the meeting.
Notice and describe the situation	Notice rather than evaluate and **describe** the situation or behaviour, without judging or blaming.	I have been off already for 6 weeks. I was hoping to return next week but there have been some complications with my recovery.

Emotions and feelings	Recognise and express how you are feeling – use 'notice and name' to label your emotions. Use 'I' statements to own your feelings.	I feel frustrated and guilty.
Ask yourself what matters most	What needs are most important to you and the other person? Aim for connection and show that you have heard what the other person has said, and you understand their perspective.	**What are my needs?** I'm really committed to the practice and being professional is really important to me. I care about my team, and I worry about them being over-stretched and short-staffed. But I also need to care for my physical health and make sure I'm recovering fully. **What might be the practice manager's needs?** He has a need for effectiveness and the practice to run smoothly, but I think he also cares about my wellbeing and wants the best for me.
Make a reasonable request	What would help to meet your important needs in this situation? Be respectful and friendly and ensure it's not a demand. Look for a strategy that meets everyone's needs and stay flexible until you reach a fair solution.	I'd like another two weeks off and to then have a slow graded return where I build up slowly to make sure I'm able to cope with my duties.

EXERCISE: Compassionate communication in action

Now it's your turn to practise using confident compassionate communication! Start with a small issue, rather than a long-standing, complex or difficult problem. Try working through the steps alone and offering yourself some empathy, before deciding what to say to the other person:

Plan and prepare	What might be a helpful time or place to have the conversation? How can you plan or prepare yourself and the other person?	

Notice and describe the situation	Notice rather than evaluate and describe the situation without judging or blaming	
Emotions and feelings	Recognise and name your feelings: "I'm feeling..."	
Ask yourself what matters most	What needs are most important to you and the other person? Aim for connection and to show that you have heard and understood the other person's perspective.	*My needs:* *The other person's needs:*
Make a reasonable request	Look for an outcome that meets everyone's needs and stay flexible until you find a mutually agreeable solution.	

Chapter summary: Connecting and communicating

- Connecting with others is essential for happiness and wellbeing.

- This may involve strengthening relationships with close friends and family and expanding your relationship circles.

- Understanding personality traits such as introversion and extroversion can help you work to your strengths and build relationships that suit your personal needs.

- If you feel anxious in a social or performance situation, try behaving 'as if' you feel just a little more confident, and shift your attention into the present moment and people around you.

- Confident compassionate communication can help you express yourself with understanding and respect, even when facing conflict or a difficult conversation.

Final thoughts

What are the most important messages for you from this chapter?

Take an action step

What are your next steps? What actions will you take as a result of reading this chapter?

What steps can you take to strengthen and build your sense of connection with those around you?

11 Surviving significant events

> - Have you been thrown off track by a major life event or an unplanned change in circumstances?
>
> - Are you struggling to recover after a significant event or a complaint, or do you feel wounded by a series of incidents and setbacks?
>
> - Are you finding it difficult to adjust to an important loss or a traumatic experience?
>
> - Reflect on these challenges and develop your personal GROWTH recovery plan. Keep reading…

11.1 Coping in hard times

We all experience stressful life events, which may arise at unexpected times or in unpredictable ways. These might include experiences at work such as a complaint, a significant event, or making a clinical error. In our personal lives, we may be coping with serious illness, financial stress, the breakdown of an important relationship, or the loss of someone close.

These events will affect us all differently, and at certain times in our lives we may feel more vulnerable or find it harder to cope. Facing a series of relatively minor challenges may have a cumulative impact, and even seemingly positive or joyful events such as moving house or having a baby can also bring high levels of stress and trigger powerful emotions. We may not always label events as a trauma but coming to terms with these experiences can be challenging and have a major impact on our emotional wellbeing.

As clinicians, we may experience traumatic events ourselves, via our family and friends, or through caring for patients and hearing their stories and experiences. Coping with these experiences involves a process of adjustment where we start to make sense of what happened and work out how to continue living and working in the face of the changes that each situation brings.

Even when we lack control over a situation, we can still influence how we respond to difficult experiences. We can take time to process these events without becoming overly preoccupied or allowing them to have a prolonged negative impact on our life and relationships with others. We can prevent incidents from creating lasting doubt about our own competence and capability.

In this chapter we will look at ways to:

- Understand your personal responses to stressful life events
- Review the impact of trauma, moral distress and moral injury
- Explore the experience of loss and grief
- Find ways to adjust and promote recovery in the face of challenging life experiences
- Develop a 'future forward plan' and summarise the **GROWTH** skills we have covered in this book.

Bridget, experienced Practice Nurse: Bridget has worked for over 20 years in her practice and is well respected by colleagues and popular with patients for her friendly, talkative manner. Since losing her partner two months ago, she has struggled to come to terms with the loss and has not yet been able to return to work.

"I'm not sleeping well and if I do drop off, I always wake up expecting to see Thomas next to me. Every morning I get a gut-wrenching reminder of the loss when he's not there. His illness was short and traumatic, and I still replay images in my mind of seeing him in the hospital bed where he died. It takes me back to my time in critical care and also when I lost my parents.

My young grandchildren keep asking where Grandad is and why he went to heaven so soon! It fills me with rage about the unfairness of it all when we were so near retirement and finally due to have some time together.

I put on my brave face but really struggle to talk to anyone about my real feelings. We did everything together and I find it hard to face the couples we used to see without feeling overwhelming guilt about still being here. I just don't feel I can deal with the outpourings of sympathy from everyone at the practice without dissolving into sobs. The thought of dealing with illness and death in my working life just feels too much at the moment."

Raj, GP Partner: Raj has been a GP for over 10 years. Last year, he became a father of twins and has been doing extra out-of-hours work to financially support his family. He became tired and stressed from trying to meet all these demands, and made a few minor mistakes at work, which were picked up by colleagues. Then he was contacted by his practice manager to inform him that a patient he had seen the previous week had died unexpectedly and that Raj would have to attend the inquest. The patient's wife also made a formal complaint about Raj's care.

"My life has been thrown completely off balance by these events. I'm finding it really difficult to keep going. There are pressures at home and my wife is exhausted as she has recently returned to work after the twins. We still don't get much sleep as one of the boys is usually awake at least once at night.

I feel so anxious and guilty about the problems at work. I can't believe I made all those silly errors – my colleagues must think I'm totally incompetent. And it has been so stressful dealing with the inquest. It involved months of stress, worry and sleepless nights. In the end, they ruled that it was an unexpected death that would have been impossible to predict.

I thought I would feel better after the inquest was over, but I don't! I'm constantly anxious and waiting for the next thing to go wrong. It affects my relationships at home, and I find it hard to concentrate and function normally at work. I'm being extra vigilant, terrified that I will make another mistake. It's like I've lost all trust in myself. I drink heavily most evenings, otherwise I'm awake all night imagining the future I worked hard for slipping away in front of me..."

11.2 Experiences of trauma

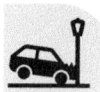

We may experience significant traumatic events within our working role or in our personal lives. These are events that are out of the ordinary, bringing an extreme sense of threat or danger, and which may trigger a trauma response. They include experiences such as:

- Serious accidents or injuries

- Physical and sexual assaults

- Childhood and domestic abuse

- Serious health problems, including intensive care admissions and childbirth

- Traumatic experiences during the pandemic, when providing care for people with Covid-19.

The trauma response

The trauma response is a normal reaction to extreme circumstances. It occurs after being exposed to a traumatic event that involves significant threat and causes feelings of intense fear, helplessness or horror.

Facing a traumatic event typically activates an acute stress reaction, via the sympathetic nervous system. The nature and severity of traumatic experiences may mean that we freeze or dissociate as coping strategies for intense feelings of fear or horror. This helps us get through the moment but may interfere with our later processing of the experience and leads to fragmented memories of the event.

The figure below gives an overview of how the CBT framework can be used to make sense of the trauma response.

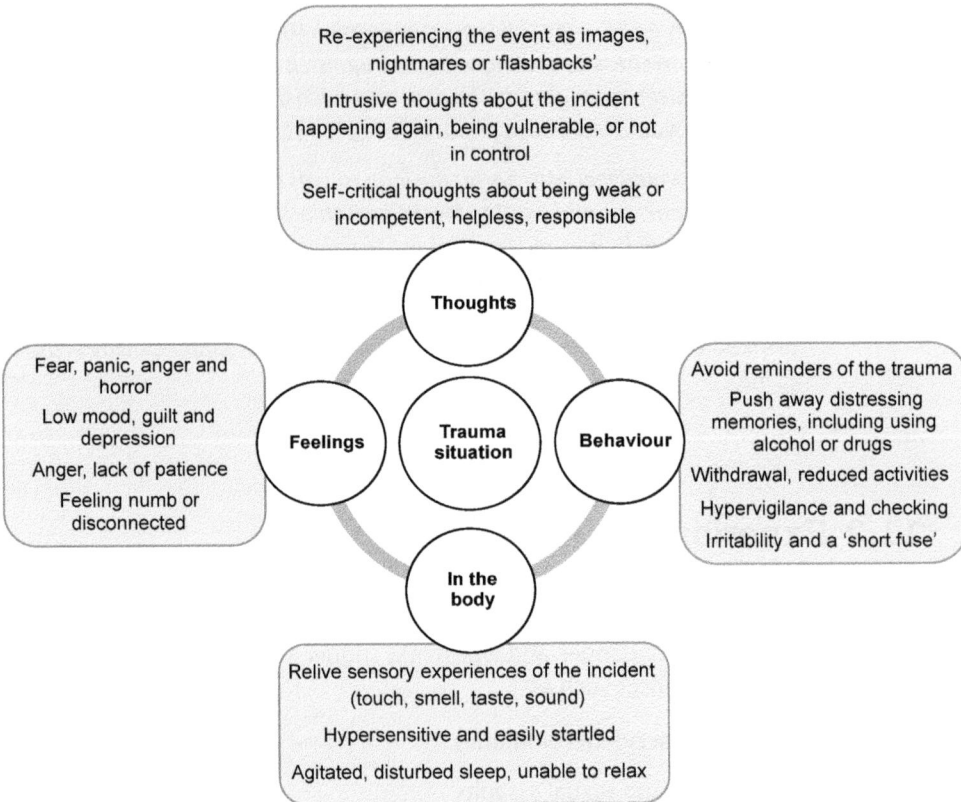

Trauma and the messy kitchen cupboard

This is a useful analogy for understanding how we process traumatic memories. If you feel extremely busy and stressed when you get home from the supermarket, you may not take time to unpack your shopping and put it away carefully. Instead, you might throw the whole bag into the cupboard as a disorganised mess, without applying logic or stacking items neatly.

Now, every time you open the cupboard door, things fall out. Even if you want to cook a meal and get on with life, you cannot find what you need. You find it stressful and distressing to know that the cupboard is so disorganised, so you stop going into the kitchen, and try to avoid thinking about it.

Over time, as you are able to process any trauma memories, it's like you have had time to come back and sort through the contents of the cupboard and organise it into food types, expiry dates and relevance. You may start to view the cupboard differently and are no longer afraid to open it. Over time, you are able to see the cupboard as part of your home, and to continue living in a meaningful way.

PAUSE AND REFLECT: Noticing trauma memories

- Have you experienced a traumatic event? This may be a single experience or a series of distressing incidents.

- Do you frequently revisit memories of the incident, or do unwanted memories come into your mind as intrusive images or disturbing thoughts?

- Complete the following table about a memory which visits you often:

Intrusive memory	Tick if this applies	When might you notice this? How often?
Unwanted thoughts about it often come into my mind		
I have nightmares or vivid dreams		
I try not to think about the memory		
I try to avoid situations that might remind me of it		
I feel watchful or easily startled		
I often feel numb or detached from others or from what I'm doing		

If you have ticked more than three or four items, you may be significantly impacted by the experience.

Post-traumatic stress disorder (PTSD)

Trauma symptoms are initially very common after a traumatic event but in most people will fade over several weeks. In 10–20%, these symptoms can persist. PTSD may be diagnosed if symptoms are severe and last longer than one month.

Factors that influence whether we may go on to develop PTSD after being exposed to trauma include having prior experiences of trauma or childhood adversity, coping with multiple life stresses, and mental health challenges. The strongest predictor for developing PTSD is a lack of social support. This emphasises the importance of turning towards others and not allowing yourself to disengage when coping with traumatic life events.

If you may have developed PTSD following a traumatic event, we strongly recommend that you attend your GP or seek other support, as you could benefit from therapy such as trauma-focused CBT or eye movement desensitisation and reprocessing (EMDR).

Self-care after trauma

The coping strategies that we turn to after a traumatic event can have a profound influence on our wellbeing and whether we experience persistent trauma symptoms.

Many clinicians fall back on the well-worn strategy of 'pushing through' and 'getting on with it' for coping with traumatic and stressful events at work. Perhaps you fear that by raising a concern or acknowledging your distress, you might 'open a can of worms' and become overwhelmed. You might also be motivated by wanting to contribute to your team and worried about appearing 'weak' or 'incompetent' in front of colleagues.

Suppressing emotion may work to an extent in the short term, and may sometimes be helpful for coping in unexpected, challenging circumstances whilst maintaining a calm professional approach. But overuse of this strategy, without taking sufficient time to emotionally process challenging events, can lead to longer-term distress and increased risk of emotional difficulties.

We can use the acronym **FACE** for some specific strategies that may help us find courage and the ability to cope after a traumatic experience:

- **F**ocus on your values and what you can control
- **A**cknowledge and allow thoughts and feelings
- **C**onnect with the people around you; offer yourself **C**ompassion for the distress
- **E**xpand your possibilities.

PAUSE AND REFLECT: Focus on your values and what you can control

Take a moment to check in with your inner **Guide** and remind yourself who and what are most important to you. Ask yourself: What do I need right now to care for myself?

Use your answers to help prioritise your actions and choices. Keep in mind values such as self-compassion, self-care and caring for others. How might you enact these following a traumatic or distressing situation? Can you plan small steps that move you towards your important values, to reduce avoidance and increase participation in meaningful and important daily activities such as work, hobbies and social interaction?

Try to focus on the aspects of life that you can control. There is little we can do about wars or disasters in other countries, but we can contribute by giving to a charity or supporting a refugee. Similarly, you may not be able to control the strong emotions that come up after experiencing trauma, but you can choose your actions, ensuring that you don't allow the experience to interfere with your relationships or ways of caring for yourself.

Acknowledge and allow

Instead of trying to suppress difficult emotions or avoid thinking about traumatic experiences, it's important to start to 'open up' or 'lean in' and acknowledge and recognise your thoughts and feelings. This can help you to step back and disentangle yourself from distressing memories and feelings.

Use **Open and Observe** skills from *Chapter 3* to notice your reactions. Is there any reluctance to accept or talk about the distressing event? Are you having intrusive thoughts or images? Trying to push these away or avoid triggering them may actually intensify their power to cause distress over time.

Instead try to notice and name your experiences with kindness and care: "I'm having a difficult memory. I'm feeling anxious and my heart is racing. This is a moment of suffering and I wish myself well as I recover from a distressing experience." You can also use grounding in your five senses to help you come back to the present moment and cope with powerful emotions without becoming overwhelmed (see *Section 3.8*).

Can you allow yourself space to acknowledge your experiences and begin to talk about it in small steps, with a close friend or partner? If talking is too difficult, try writing in a journal or speaking into a voice recorder – anything to start to open up to what has happened and create space to process your experiences.

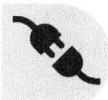

Connect with people around you and offer yourself compassion for the distress

Connecting with important colleagues, friends and family is an essential step to gain support and inner resources to cope after a traumatic experience. You may feel an urge to isolate yourself from colleagues, friends and family. However, this often increases anxiety and the sense of threat, and may also lower your mood as you disengage from people you care about.

You may find that you need to talk repetitively about the trauma, and this can be helpful to slowly process and make sense of an incomprehensible experience. If you don't feel like talking, you might prefer to spend quiet time with others at first. It can be comforting to know you're not alone.

Balancing your threat–drive system with soothing is vital to reduce hypervigilance and tension. Mindfulness, relaxation and paying attention to soothing touch or taste can all aid with sleep and reduce physical tension.

Self-compassion can help to manage feelings of guilt and shame, which are common after experiencing trauma. This can take many different forms, such as drinking your favourite tea, winding down with a hot bath, listening to music, or hiking to a beautiful viewpoint with friends.

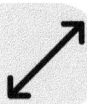

Expand your possibilities and explore alternative options

Wise Mind can help you re-frame self-critical or catastrophic thoughts, become less reactive, and expand your perspective. Pause and notice your daily routines or patterns of behaviour – how helpful are these? Can you find some ways to expand your choices and promote positive self-care and healthy life habits, such as physical exercise, sleep hygiene and healthy eating? You may also benefit from cutting back from unhealthy choices such as excessive alcohol.

Encourage acceptance of what has happened and try to notice any small things you can appreciate in the present moment. Take a look out of the window or up at the sky and engage with your five senses as you appreciate your surroundings and ground yourself in the here and now.

Raj reflects: *"I'm still struggling a lot with anxiety so I referred myself to NHS Practitioner Health. It was helpful to have an appointment with a clinician with plenty of time to go over all my concerns and get some perspective. We agreed that I would start CBT for anxiety, and if I'm still struggling, I'm willing to consider antidepressant medication. I'd prefer not to, but it's good to have a greater sense of control and choice about how I feel.*

I realised that I've been using a lot of unhelpful ways to try and suppress traumatic memories about the problems I've been facing. A big one is that I've started drinking quite heavily, and in the mornings I often feel tired and a little hungover. I can see that this is an 'away step' – it disconnects me from my family and makes it harder to function at work the next day. I'm going to make a big effort to cut down alcohol – as well as the 6 coffees I often drink the next day! And instead, spend more quality time with my family. Maybe I will restart a hobby – I used to really enjoy playing board games – I might get a couple down from the loft and we can play as a family or watch a movie together."

Find a safe place

Can you find a physical place where you feel calm and soothed, and have time to pause and process a difficult experience? It might be a garden, a woodland or curled up on your sofa. You can also create an imaginary safe space in your own mind:

Imagine a place that feels safe, peaceful and a refuge for you. We will use our five senses to explore this place:

- What can you see? Are you in a peaceful forest, looking down from a high mountain, by a lake, or staring out to sea on a beautiful beach?

- What can you hear? Can you hear the gentle sea breeze, the rhythmic sounds of the sea, rustling branches, birdsong, water rippling or calming music?

- What can you smell? Is there the salty smell of sea air, fresh mown grass, gentle scent of flower blossom?

- What can you touch around you? Can you feel the sun warming your face, the wind blowing through your hair, or the warm sand under your feet, or the rough bark of a tree?

- Emotions: how does it feel to be in this safe place? Is it possible to allow yourself to let go of any tension?

- Allow any pleasant feelings to stay with you and let the image gently fade. Then return your attention to the present moment. Remember that you can come back here at any time. This is a space just for you.

11.3 Loss and grief

Coping with loss is an inevitable part of life. Grief is not an illness or a mental health disorder but is a natural part of healing and recovery after an important loss. Nevertheless, periods of grief can bring some of the most difficult times in a person's life. We may experience grief when faced by many different types of loss, including:

- Death of a family member, close friend or colleague or a loved pet

- Breakdown or loss of an important relationship

- Ill health, or physical changes in our body from illness or surgery

- Losing an important role, such as after retirement or when children leave home

- Loss of financial or emotional security or relocation from a familiar environment

- Coping with any major life change, especially if unwanted or unexpected.

Grief emotions

Grief can involve many different emotions, including sadness, anger, fear, worry and guilt. At times we might also feel numb or disconnected from our feelings. Physical reactions are also common, including loss of appetite, headache, nausea and abdominal pain.

Some feelings experienced in grief include:

Anxiety: experiencing a significant loss may trigger anxiety about our human vulnerability and the unpredictability and fragility of life. We may start fearing that danger is around every corner, and we feel constantly on edge, with physical symptoms such as a racing heart and muscle tension.

Anger: this may be directed towards specific individuals or groups such as authority figures or organisations. We may also feel anger towards ourselves for past actions or mistakes which may have contributed to the loss.

Guilt: thoughts such as 'I should have done more' or 'I should have been able to prevent this' can trigger strong feelings of guilt. We may also feel guilt and self-criticism about our response to the loss, with thoughts such as: 'I'm weak, I'm not handling it well. I should be over this by now!'

The grief journey

There are many different ways to understand the process of grieving.

Stages of grief

You may be familiar with Kübler-Ross's 'stages of grief' model, which describes five stages (see figure below). These can be useful for understanding some of the different reactions we might have to a significant loss.

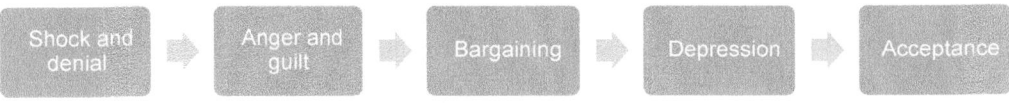

But it's also important to remember that every grief journey is unique. The stages will not arise in any specific order, and you may switch between stages at different times. You may experience a range of other reactions and emotions and may not experience some of these stages at all.

The dual process model of grief

The dual process model of grief (Stroebe and Schut, 1999) suggests that we may go back and forth or 'oscillate' between two ways of coping with grief (see figure below).

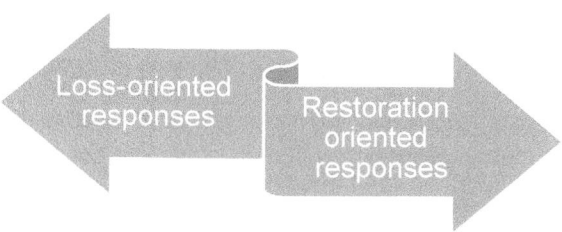

- **Loss-oriented responses:** these are thoughts, feelings, actions and events that focus on your grief and pain. It might involve thinking about how much you miss the person, looking at old photos, or bringing to mind particular memories. This is often associated with powerful emotions, such as sadness, loneliness and anger.

- **Restoration-oriented responses:** here, you engage in activities that distract you from your grief and allow you to continue with daily life. This helps to ease emotional distress for a short while, and allows you to carry out important practical tasks, plans and responsibilities.

For many people, it can be helpful to know that it is a normal and healthy part of the grief process to oscillate between these two coping responses. This can also enable us to tackle the reality of a major loss in small steps as we move in and out of intense grief.

The task-based model of grief

The task-based model (Worden, 2009) describes four 'tasks' of healthy grief:

- To accept the reality of the loss: moving from shock or disbelief towards acceptance of the loss. Rituals such as funerals and memorial services can help.

- To experience and process the pain of loss: this involves facilitating the safe expression of all our natural grief reactions.

- To adapt and adjust to a world that includes the loss or change.

- To slowly move forwards as we re-invest in a different reality and new ways of living.

Prolonged and traumatic grief

A variety of factors and circumstances can influence our experience of loss and may interfere with the grief process. These include:

- Whether a loss was expected or sudden

- Circumstances such as death by suicide, natural disaster or human violence

- Experiencing conflict associated with the loss or change

- Whether you were involved in the process of change or able to say goodbye

- The support you had around during and after the loss.

If you are experiencing prolonged grief, which persists for more than 6 months after the loss, you may benefit from talking therapy such as counselling or CBT.

Some losses can be extremely distressing and may even trigger a trauma reaction. You might experience repeated distressing unwanted images, such as flashbacks or nightmares, and you may benefit from specific therapy such as trauma-focused CBT or EMDR.

Coping with loss

Sometimes just having information and developing self-understanding that makes sense of your own responses to grief and loss, can help you to see it as a necessary process which is common to all of us. Simply recognising that a challenging experience involves some form of loss and grief may be extremely helpful.

Facing retirement is really affecting me. I think this is grief for an important loss.

We can also use **GROWTH** skills to support us during the grief journey.

Follow your inner Guide

When feeling overwhelmed by a powerful grief reaction, anchor yourself by focusing on important values such as kindness, support, connection with others and self-care. As you follow your inner **Guide**, you may find ways to recognise and attend to your needs and retain a sense of what is still important to you, even following a significant loss. Slowly and gently try to find your sense of meaning and purpose and appreciate what is still here, in your life and in your future. There's no need to force this – it often takes time to adjust and adapt to loss and change.

Ready for action – active steps for self-care

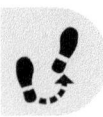

When coping with grief it's often helpful to reduce your activities and pressures for a while, saying no to unnecessary demands, reducing your workload and choosing activities that are restful, soothing and energising. Try to establish a flexible routine which finds a balance between 'mourning activities' which help you to adapt to the loss, and 'restorative activities' that allow time and space for recovery. Think about what activities you used to enjoy before the loss. Do you feel ready to start these again?

Getting support from others is extremely important when coping with loss. People may be more understanding than we expect, and often wish to help but may not know how. Try to think about what type of support would benefit you most at different times. Sometimes you might need a supportive space to express your emotions freely about the loss. At other times, you might benefit from practical support or in ways that create a distraction or respite from strong grief emotions.

Support groups can also be helpful, either in person or online. These can reduce the sense of isolation that you may feel after a loss, especially in challenging situations, such as a traumatic bereavement.

EXERCISE: Planning self-care steps

Use the following table to choose activities that might support you:

Type of activity	Examples	What might you try? Who might you reach out to for support with this?
Mourning activities: remembering and talking about the loss, enabling you to connect with and process your grief emotions	Visiting a special place, looking at old photos, or listening to music that reminds you of the person. Talking aloud to the person you have lost and imagining their responses.	
Restful activities: keep you focused on the present and absorb your attention to give you a break from the work of mourning	Sport or exercise, knitting or cooking, researching interests and hobbies. Time alone walking or gardening. Travelling or exploring.	
Seeking connection and support: turning towards friends and family to help air your thoughts, process your emotions, and find practical help	Reaching out to close family and friends. Seeking practical support with tasks such as childcare, probate, clearing out personal items, or household tasks.	

Open and Observe

The process of grief may get 'stuck' if we try to avoid our feelings about the loss or become too immersed in the loss. Try not to isolate yourself due to fears that your emotions will be overwhelming, out of control, or a source of embarrassment or shame.

Strong emotions may come in waves, often seemingly out of nowhere. You can create some space and time to sit with these and allow them to pass. Try to notice, name, normalise and validate the painful experiences that arise during the process of grief. You can use many of the **Open and Observe** skills from *Chapter 3*, such as being able to notice the NOW and connect with your five senses.

Mourning is an ongoing process which involves reflecting and processing over a period of time. There may be aspects of your loss that can never be explained. But we can live better with the uncertainty of unanswered questions when we have space and opportunity to talk it through and piece the story together with those around us.

When you are talking about the loss, remember to periodically 'check in' with yourself and make room for your experiences. Pause in the flow of words and notice: How am I feeling? What's happening in my body? What thoughts or memories are coming up?

Use Wise Mind

Loss is universal and it can be helpful to gain perspective and a sense of belonging, recognising that you are not alone in this experience.

Notice if you are having any demanding or critical thoughts such as: "I should be able to cope better than this. I'm being weak." These can lead to behaviour such as pushing through or ignoring your feelings and needs, which can get in the way of processing your grief.

Instead, can you use kind self-talk? This involves using language that is supportive and has a friendly tone. When hit by a wave of grief, you might say something like: "This is a painful moment – it really hurts. There's a huge sense of loss. This is grief, and it's really hard. I'd like to be kind to myself."

It's helpful to remember the loss in a balanced way that includes both positive experiences and any difficulties or flaws. When we idealise our past memories, we may get stuck, unable to mourn for a fully dimensional person, with all their strengths and weaknesses. Similarly, if you experienced conflict with someone, after their loss you may focus on feelings of anger and resentment. Here, you could benefit from recognising their positive qualities and acknowledging feelings such as sadness or loss, as you slowly make sense of your complex relationship with the person you lost.

EXERCISE: Using Wise Mind to pay your respects

In this exercise we will bring to mind three memories relating to an experience of loss. You could write these down or talk about them with someone you trust.

- **A neutral memory:** first, bring to mind an everyday memory or image of the person or loss that you are experiencing. You might imagine the person eating breakfast, working at the computer, or driving a car. Choose an example that doesn't bring strong emotions.

- **A negative memory:** now bring to mind a memory that is more challenging but is not highly distressing or overwhelming. Can you remember a time that the person lost their temper, behaved badly, or caused you frustration, annoyance or distress?

- **A positive memory:** finally bring to mind a positive memory associated with your loss. This might be a special time you had together, or a time that they demonstrated their best qualities.

Pause and reflect: what's the impact of taking a balanced view of the loss that takes into account neutral, difficult, and positive aspects of your loss?

Raj reflects: *"I thought I was mainly coping with stress and worry, but I've realised that under my anxiety there is also a big sense of loss. I've lost a lot of my sense of certainty and trust in myself and the world. It felt like things were stable and now they are no longer safe. I've been really struggling to come to terms with it. I've felt a lot of blame and anger towards myself and the world for allowing this to happen. It just doesn't seem fair.*

There are no quick fixes for how I feel, but even recognising the loss does feel helpful, like I'm being heard and understood a bit more. I'm trying to bring in my Wise Mind and find a wider perspective – I know I'm not the only clinician this has happened to. And I also know that I'm doing my best – I'm only human and I can't expect myself to be perfect. I'm trying to use kinder self-talk and use self-compassion rather than self-criticism…"

Thrive and Balance

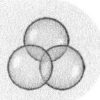

Keeping your emotion systems in balance can be difficult during the grief process, and it's normal for emotions to change rapidly and unpredictably. Your goal is not to suppress your feelings but to find ways to support yourself through each wave of emotion.

It can help to engage your calm and connect system (see *Section 5.6*) and find a sense of self-compassion. How might a wise and caring supporter offer understanding and comfort to help you cope with the pain of the loss? What would you say to a colleague, friend or patient in a similar situation?

Are there any small ways that you could show yourself care? Try one of the following:

- Friendly self-touch: place a hand over your heart, give yourself a hug, or place a hand over where the discomfort arises, and send yourself a sense of comfort or kindness.

- Supportive imagery: imagine a kindly or supportive figure, notice the kind expression in their eyes, or imagine wrapping yourself in a warm, soft blanket.

- Kind actions: plan actions based on kindness, compassion and self-understanding. Can you give yourself permission to let go of certain demands for a while, or to spend time with supportive people?

- Use a comforting object: choose something that feels good against your skin, such as a soft pillow, or stroke the fur of a soft blanket or a pet that you care about.

Healthy Life Habits

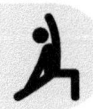

Grief can cause us to neglect our health or use drugs or alcohol to avoid or numb the pain of loss. You may be adjusting to significant changes in your role or your patterns of living, which can throw your regular routines and healthy habits off course. If you have lost a caring role, or are adjusting to retirement, you may have more time than before, or a sense of lack of purpose. Finding meaningful ways to direct your energy and looking after yourself can feel very challenging.

Creating a realistic routine that isn't excessively demanding can be a helpful way of coping with loss. This helps provide some structure in your day at a time when life may feel unpredictable or out of control. It can help you to re-engage with activities that are in line with your inner **Guide**, bringing a sense of meaning and purpose back to life. Planning your routine in advance can also reduce the burden of constant daily decision-making which may feel exhausting and draining.

Keep to the basics: Eat, Move, Sleep, Repeat. Try to plan regular mealtimes and ensure you are taking care of your physical needs for nutrition. You might struggle with your appetite and may find that simple small meals are easier to manage. Ensuring that you eat with someone or go out to eat several times in the week can also help.

If you are struggling with sleep, follow some of our advice in *Section 6.6* about creating a bedtime routine, including taking time to wind down before bed with a soothing activity.

Exercise is a helpful way to maintain wellbeing when grieving. This might involve going for walks, or something more physically active such as running or swimming. Try starting with regular short amounts of low intensity activity, picking something that you find restful or energising.

Bridget reflects: *"Losing Thomas has been one of the hardest things I've had to cope with. I think I need to give myself permission to find it difficult. I've been giving myself a hard time for not getting over it more quickly, and I'm starting to recognise that I need to allow myself more time to grieve. I'm not ready to go back to work yet. I spoke to my GP, who was very kind, and I told the practice manager yesterday. She was incredibly supportive – sending condolences and love from the whole practice team – and even the phone call made me quite tearful.*

I can see that I've been pulling away from people because I didn't want to overwhelm them with my emotions – but I'm also realising that others really do want to help. I've been making the effort to see my son and my grandchildren more regularly – they are probably the most important people in my life now. And I'm trying to answer their questions about Grandad honestly – acknowledging how we all miss him so very much.

I've reached out to my oldest friend Carmen who lives round the corner. She's offered to help me make a start with going through some of Thomas's things and to do some of the admin that Thomas always used to take care of. I like the idea of oscillating in and out of grief – sometimes I'm a sobbing wreck and other times Carmen and I can have a laugh together – and I don't have to feel guilty about finding some laughter amidst the grief. I even got back to my Zumba class this week – it felt good to hear the music and move my body a bit. I'm focusing on taking small steps and trying to be kinder to myself on the way."

Processing through writing

Journaling can help us to process loss and experiences of trauma through writing. Write down as much detail as possible, using the following prompts:

- Describe the time leading up to the incident, trauma or loss.

- What were the circumstances? What important events occurred during the experience?

- Reflect on the time following the loss or trauma. If you are writing about a bereavement, include mourning activities such as a funeral or memorial service. For an injury or trauma, describe your injuries, rehabilitation and recovery process.

- Notice if any part of the story feels particularly emotionally charged, or 'stuck'. Is anything particularly hard to accept or understand, or are there unanswered questions or areas of conflict? Is there any way to make sense of these or can you offer yourself compassion for any distress that you experience?

- Ask yourself the following questions as you write:
    - what images or pictures come to mind?
    - what thoughts are most difficult?
    - what emotions or body sensations come up?
    - how can I be kind and offer myself support?
- Consider including other people's perspectives and emotional responses to the loss or trauma, which may help you to make sense of your own experience.

11.4 Moral distress and injury

Moral distress is a feeling of psychological unease that arises when we need to behave in ways that conflict with our personal beliefs or morals, especially when we perceive this as avoidable, or feel powerless to change it. It may arise when we feel unable to provide the level of care that we wish to, perhaps due to insufficient staff, resources, referral pathways or time. Moral distress can also arise when we feel betrayed by others including leaders, politicians and the wider health service.

Moral injury can occur if sustained moral distress leads to impaired function or longer-term psychological harm. Moral injury can produce profound guilt or shame, as well as feelings of betrayal and anger, and increases the risk of conditions such as PTSD and depression.

PAUSE AND REFLECT: Noticing moral distress

Have you experienced a sense of moral distress?

- What was the situation? Who and what was involved in this reaction?
- What was the impact on you? What thoughts, feelings or behaviours did you notice?

Coping with moral distress and injury

Managing moral distress and injury often involves organisational changes that create a fundamental platform for wellbeing in healthcare staff. These include adequate funding and resourcing, appropriate levels of staffing, developing an open culture in the workplace, and providing support and empowerment for clinicians. We may not always have the ability to influence or control this.

Health professionals can also use self-care skills to protect themselves, and many of the skills for coping after grief and trauma can be applied to managing moral distress. Some extra steps include:

- Talking openly about moral distress and its impact within your team

- Strengthening support within your team and actively seeking advice from colleagues

- Focusing on meaning and purpose at work

- Noticing personality traits such as being a chronic hero or an imposter, which may mean you struggle with guilt and personal responsibility or set yourself unreachable expectations or targets (see *Chapter 7*)

- Actively finding ways to bring self-care into your work and home life.

Raj reflects: *"Moral distress could explain why I felt so anxious, even after the inquest was over. I felt really fed up and disillusioned with the system for putting me through so much stress, even when I didn't actually make a major error. I feel extremely frustrated with the current impossible demand for appointments and being unable to see everyone face-to-face. It seems like we are being set up for things to go wrong.*

It feels quite a relief to recognise this. I know I can be a bit of a chronic hero, and this case brought out a huge sense of guilt and personal responsibility. Plus, my imposter beliefs meant that I was concealing how I felt from colleagues.

Lately, I've been trying to talk a bit more openly about moral distress, in the coffee room and at practice meetings. And instead of struggling in silence, I've been trying to turn to colleagues for support. My team have been great – and it's helpful to hear more about other people's struggles and challenges and realise I'm not alone in finding general practice hard. I know I need to work on my self-care. I'm going to try mindfulness, and maybe get my bike out of the garage and go for a ride with my brother, who is an avid cyclist."

Chapter summary: Surviving significant events

Experiences of loss and significant life events including trauma are common to us all and may be a source of anxiety, grief and emotional distress. Skills for coping include:

- Following your inner **Guide** to re-establish your sense of meaning and purpose

- Maintaining a flexible reasonable routine, regular activity and realistic goals

- Connecting and seeking support from others, rather than slipping into isolation or avoidance

- Using **Open and Observe** to pause and make space for difficult emotions, allowing them to pass naturally in their own time

- Using **Wise Mind** to find perspective and use kind self-talk that acknowledges and offers a caring response to your distress

- Balancing your emotion systems, finding ways to develop self-soothing and self-compassion.

- Choosing **Healthy Life Habits** that encourage self-care, including physical activity, sleep and healthy eating.

Final thoughts

What are the most important messages for you from this chapter?

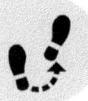

Take an action step

What are your next steps? What actions will you take as a result of reading this chapter?

What steps can you take to strengthen your resources to cope with stressful, distressing or traumatic events?

12 Putting it all together

- Did you start this book with hopeful intentions then other demands took over?

- Have you managed to make some helpful changes and wonder if this will last?

- Are you already criticising yourself for not making enough changes? Keep reading…

12.1 Where are you now?

This is not the beginning, nor the end…. It is the end of the beginning….

We started this book with the acknowledgement that working in primary care and the wider health service can be hugely rewarding but may also be difficult, demanding and demoralising. Change is constant, driven by forces beyond our control such as funding, government policies and new contracts. We need to adapt to new ways of working whilst coping with stresses arising from negative or hostile attitudes towards health professionals.

Coping with these challenges requires emotional strength, flexibility and resilience, and can be achieved using the **GROWTH** steps that we have introduced throughout this book. You may already have started to include these in your daily life in small ways. The next step is to continue and build on this progress in ways that benefit you personally.

Of course, sometimes 'life happens'. Perhaps there is a new priority or an unexpected problem that demands your time and attention. You may find that you've lost focus on your positive new habits or allowed them to slide. This is completely normal and it's important not to jump into self-criticism or blame, which might make it harder to pick them up again.

Determination, resilience and self-compassion are essential tools to reflect on what's happened, and what the next helpful step might be. As with any new skill, we need to keep practicing, revising, and refining our knowledge and actions in order to make it a healthy habit. This may involve switching off the critic that tells you that you have not done enough and bringing on the coach to acknowledge and praise whatever small step you have taken in the direction of what matters most.

12.2 Recapping the GROWTH steps

Meaningful and lasting skill development is achieved by practice and repetition. We have encouraged you throughout this book to try things out, write them down, practise and repeat them to create healthy habits.

Use the following table to reflect on the **GROWTH** steps we have introduced through the book, and how you might continue to use these to understand yourself and support your wellbeing.

Guide: follow your inner Guide to identify meaningful activities linked to your values and needs. Show gratitude and appreciation for things that matter to you most.	**The things that bring meaning and purpose to my life and which I am grateful for are…**
Ready for Action: set some goals, linked to your values, which add SPICE to your life, energise you and boost your mood. Create a clear plan which involves realistic small steps.	**My immediate goals and plans are…**
Open and Observe: notice any negative thought patterns and the impact on your mood. Use mindfulness and observe skills to step back and stop yourself getting caught up by worry, rumination or distressing feelings. Engage with your senses or a valued activity to help move forwards.	**My negative thoughts or 'mind visitors' are…** **Uncomfortable feelings that come up for me include…** **The Open and Observe skills I will practise are…**

Wise Mind: choose which thoughts to listen to and which actions will provide the best outcome for you. What is the perspective of your Wise inner coach or supporter?	**My Wise perspective is…** **How would I advise or support a colleague or friend?** **My Wise or supportive coach would say…**
Thrive and Balance: is your threat system overloaded with stressors that could be dealt with using problem-solving? Keep a balance by activating your drive and calm and connect systems.	**The stressors I can problem-solve and reduce are…** **I will balance my emotion system by…**
Healthy Life Habits: keep up important wellbeing habits such as eating regular healthy meals, physical activity and sleep.	**I will maintain healthy habits by…**

12.3 Future forward plan

Finally, complete this 'future forward plan' which can remind you what you have learnt so far, and help you make a plan of your next steps for the future.

The most useful things I have learnt about myself are:

The most useful GROWTH skills and techniques I have learnt are:

What changes have I made? What am I doing differently?

What's next? How can I build on this? What changes can I continue to make over the next 6–12 months?

What could be a sign that I'm slipping back into unwanted habits?

What would be a helpful way to respond if I notice things are becoming more difficult? What can I do? Who can I ask for help?

Glossary of key terms

Here is a summary list of the main terms and techniques we have covered throughout this book:

ABLE model of uncertainty: this is a four-step approach to help you cope when struggling with any kind of uncertainty:

- **A**cknowledge and **A**llow

- **B**reathe

- **L**abel your experiences and **L**et go of the need for certainty

- **E**xpand your attention and come back to doing something important.

ACCEPTS model of uncertainty: this model gives some helpful steps for health professionals to manage uncertainty:

- **A**cknowledge and **A**llow uncertainty

- **C**linical knowledge and judgement

- **C**ommunicate effectively

- **E**ngage in helpful behaviour

- **P**artnership and **P**ractice teams

- **T**est of time

- **S**elf-compassion.

Action spoilers: these are examples of common types of Away actions such as fear, anger, fatigue, procrastination and self-critical thoughts, or negative predictions about what may go wrong.

Activity diary: this is a way of recording your activities over each day or week to identify helpful and unhelpful patterns of behaviour.

Anxiety alarm system: it can be helpful to view anxiety as a type of alarm or warning system. It may be a little too sensitive if you tend to over-estimate or exaggerate the risks in your mind, but it's an important system that cannot be removed or eliminated.

Anxiety mind visitors: these are negative thoughts that are common in anxiety, such as tending to exaggerate the risks, focus on what could go wrong, imagine that you can't cope, and seeking excessive certainty.

ARC: this is a strategy to help you create a bridge over difficult experiences and move towards where you wish to go:

- Acknowledge the thought and feeling

- Recognise the urge to react

- Choose your Wise response

Autopilot: when you carry out habitual actions without paying full attention to what you are doing.

Away actions: behaviours that move you away from your values and sense of purpose, usually because you are trying to reduce difficult feelings or distress.

Big picture perspective: this involves finding some distance and perspective which takes into account your wider values, knowledge and wisdom about the world.

Boom–bust activity patterns: this involves over-exertion and exhaustion followed by prolonged rest. It can lead to physical deconditioning and worsens symptoms such as fatigue and pain. A more helpful approach involves making gradual changes in activity and trying not to stop completely when facing setbacks.

CBT framework: use the five areas of the CBT framework to map out and understand your responses to difficult experiences:

- Thoughts, beliefs and thinking patterns

- Feelings and emotions

- Physical reactions in the body

- Behaviour, actions and urges

- Situation, environment and triggers.

Chronic hero: this personality trait is common in health professionals who are often compassionate, caring individuals, but may also struggle with excessive guilt and an exaggerated sense of duty and personal responsibility, even for things that are outside their control.

Confident compassionate communication: this involves four steps, which call for getting NEAR to others:

- **N**otice and describe the situation without judgement

- **E**motions: recognise and express how you are feeling

- **A**sk yourself what matters most (to you and the other person)

- **R**easonable request – what might help meet your/their needs?

Defuse from unhelpful thoughts: cognitive defusion involves stepping back and noticing any thoughts that show up, whilst also recognising that they are just thoughts, not absolute fact.

FACE hard times: this is an acronym for some specific strategies to help us find courage and the ability to cope after a traumatic or difficult experience:

- **F**ocus on your values and what you can control

- **A**cknowledge and allow thoughts and feelings

- **C**onnect with the people around you and offer yourself **C**ompassion

- **E**xpand your possibilities.

Five senses: if you are overwhelmed by thoughts and feelings, you can use your five senses to ground yourself in the moment:

- What can you see around you?

- What sounds can you hear?

- What are you touching with your hands or skin?

- What can you smell or taste?

- Are there any sensations inside your body?

- What's going through your mind?

- Finish by breathing out slowly with a long gentle sigh and connect with what's most important for you to be doing at this moment.

Flexible attention: enables you to observe, move and shift your focus of attention, helping you to remain aware of the present moment and avoid getting 'hooked' by negative thoughts or over-focused on a task.

Flow: a state of heightened concentration and focus when you are fully absorbed by a task or activity, which brings feelings of contentment and satisfaction.

Gratitude and appreciation: this involves actively paying attention to any small positive life experience, or things that have gone well, or things in your life that you appreciate, rather than only focusing on things that go wrong.

Habits: repeated behaviours which you carry out regularly, which may be helpful or unhelpful in the wider context of your life.

Healthy life habits: these are patterns of behaviour that support emotional and physical wellbeing, including being physically active, having healthy eating patterns, getting enough sleep, and caring for your physical health.

High road: a neurological pathway which involves processing information in higher areas of the brain, such as the prefrontal cortex. Instead of triggering the stress response, the 'high road' pathways enable you to reflect, gain perspective, and take a more realistic and thoughtful response to challenging situations.

Imposter syndrome: people with this personality trait are often highly successful but experience persistent self-doubt about their own abilities, and constantly fear being exposed as a 'fraud'.

Inner Guide: your internal compass which points towards your personal values.

Life-boosting actions: these bring a sense of enjoyment, achievement or satisfaction, and are important and meaningful to you.

Life-draining actions: behaviours which lower your mood or energy levels, and don't add value to your life.

Low mood swamp: feeling low can feel like getting stuck in a giant swamp. Feeling exhausted, low and demoralised all make it harder to take positive action, but doing less makes you sink even deeper. The route out of the swamp involves taking small steps towards a meaningful activity by behaving 'as if' you feel slightly better.

Low road: a neurological pathway in the brain which triggers the threat response and the sympathetic 'fight, flight or freeze' response.

Micro-steps: these involve tiny behavioural changes which can help to break ingrained habits and create a positive cycle that leads to improvement over time.

Mind visitors: these are patterns of negative thinking that often pop up or 'pay a visit' to your mind, and may trigger negative emotions such as low mood or anxiety.

Mind worms: these represent intrusive thoughts and inner conversations that spiral round repeatedly in your mind, such as self-critical recriminations or worry about future problems.

Moral distress and injury: this is a feeling of psychological unease which may arise when we need to work or behave in ways that conflict with our personal beliefs or morals, especially when we perceive this as avoidable, or feel powerless to change it.

NAME your values and needs: a four-step process for recognising what's most important to you:

- **N**otice your value or need
- **A**llow yourself space to pause and ground yourself in the present moment, using your five senses
- **A**sk yourself what matters most?
- **E**ngage in a valued activity with your full attention.

Needs: the immediate urges or impulses that affect you in the context of a particular situation.

Notice the NOW: a useful technique for when your mind wanders or you are becoming preoccupied with negative thoughts and feelings:

- **N**otice and name your thoughts and feelings

- **O**bserve your outer body and the world around, using your five senses

- **W**hat matters? Decide what's most important to focus on and move to do this with your full attention.

Obsessional focus: people with this personality trait are typically hard-working, reliable and conscientious, but also tend to prioritise work over relationships, and get so caught up in rules and schedules that they lose the purpose of what they are doing or cause difficulties in relationships with other people.

Open and Observe: stepping back and becoming aware of what's happening in your body and mind and in the world around, and being able to notice and acknowledge your thoughts, feelings and urges without judgement or getting caught up in them.

Rapid relief: this is a strategy we may try in order to rapidly alleviate emotional distress or discomfort, often by seeking reassurance, avoidance or trying to be absolutely certain. These actions may lead to a short-term reduction in difficult feelings but the relief is only temporary and usually worsens distress in the long term.

Ready to take action: concrete actions and behaviours that you consciously choose to take, including preparing for change.

Relationship circles: we have many different types of relationships in our lives, which vary in how close you feel and how well you know the other person. These include close family, supporters, wider friends and colleagues, and acquaintances.

Responsibility pie chart: this can help you take a more objective and realistic perspective when you are struggling with excessive guilt, blame or responsibility:

- Describe the situation or event that you are taking responsibility for.

- List the people/places/organisations/situations involved. Include yourself last on the list.

- Draw a circle and allocate a slice of 'pie' to each person according to how much responsibility and control they have. Fit your own slice in last.

- Reflect on any change in perspective and decide on helpful next steps.

Rumination: this involves thinking repeatedly over a problem or past event where something has gone wrong, and is common in low mood.

Self-compassion: this involves offering yourself kindness, acceptance and understanding, rather than slipping into self-criticism, judgement or blame when facing problems or difficulties.

SPICE activities: this is an acronym for different types of activity that may lead to a lift in low mood. Choose activities that involve one or more of the following:

- **S**uccess or achievement
- **P**hysical activity
- **I**mportant and meaningful
- **C**onnection or closeness
- **E**njoyable, relaxing and fun.

Stress bucket: this is a way of imagining stress as like water flowing into a bucket. To prevent it from overflowing you can:

- Reduce pressures and demands (flow into the bucket)
- Develop your coping strategies (improve drainage from the bucket)
- Increase the size or flexibility of the bucket using self-compassion and by seeking support.

Supportive coach: you can learn to treat yourself like a supportive coach or mentor who motivates with encouragement, kindness and wisdom, rather than blame or criticism.

Thinking time: this is a strategy for coping with excessive worry. You plan a regular convenient time to reflect and think about your problems without spending the whole day constantly worrying.

Thinking trap: common patterns of thoughts that can pull you into seeing the world in a negative way, such as negative bias, catastrophising, excessive doubt, perfectionism and self-criticism.

Thrive and Balance your three circles of emotion: keep a balance between these systems to avoid overwhelm:

- Threat system: for survival and self-protection, mediated by sympathetic nervous system
- Drive system: to motivate us to seek out what we want and need; dopamine release triggers a rush of excitement when you achieve your goals
- Calm and connect system: enables you to respond to emotional distress and to give and receive support and care from others.

Towards actions: behaviours which are in line with your values and needs, the life you wish to lead and the person you wish to be. We can carry out a Towards step even in the presence of uncomfortable thoughts and feelings.

Unhealthy perfectionism: this personality trait involves relentlessly pursuing demanding or unreasonably high standards which are impossible to achieve in the real world, and basing your self-worth on achieving them.

Values: your long-term priorities about the people and activities that matter most, giving your life meaning and purpose.

Wise Mind: engaging your **Wise Mind** involves balancing logic and emotions, looking at the big picture and thinking flexibly, adapting your perspective to meet new challenges and looking for ways to solve problems.

Worry decision tree: this involves deciding whether a worry is something you have some control over and can take action to resolve, or whether it's something that is outside your control.

References and further reading

Bennett, R. and Oliver, J. (2019) *Acceptance and Commitment Therapy: 100 key points and techniques*. Routledge.

Blackwelder, R., Hood Watson, K. and Freedy, J.R. (2016) Physician wellness across the professional spectrum. *Primary Care*, **43(2):** 355–61.

Bourne, T., Vanderhaegen, J., Vranken, R. *et al.* (2016) Doctors' experiences and their perception of the most stressful aspects of complaints processes in the UK: an analysis of qualitative survey data. *BMJ Open*, **6(7):** 1–10.

Brabban, A. and Turkington, D. (2002) 'The search for meaning: detecting congruence between life events, underlying schema and psychotic symptoms'. In A.P. Morrison (ed.) *A Casebook of Cognitive Therapy for Psychosis* (pp. 59–75). Brunner-Routledge.

British Medical Association (2015) *National Survey of GPs: the future of general practice*. BMA.

British Medical Association (2019) *Mental Health and Wellbeing in the Medical Profession*. BMA.

British Medical Association (2021) *Moral distress and moral injury: recognising and tackling it for UK doctors*. BMA.

David, L. (2013) *Using CBT in General Practice: the 10 minute consultation*, 2nd edition. Scion Publishing.

Gazelle, G., Liebschutz, J.M. and Riess, H. (2015) Physician burnout: coaching a way out. *J Gen Intern Med*, **30(4):** 508–13.

Gilbert, P. (2010) *Compassion Focused Therapy: distinctive features*. Routledge.

Greenberger, D. and Padesky, C.A. (2015) *Mind Over Mood: change how you feel by changing the way you think*. Guilford Press.

Harris, R. (2019) *ACT Made Simple: an easy-to-read primer on acceptance and commitment therapy*, 2nd edition. New Harbinger.

Harris, R. (2022) *The Happiness Trap: how to stop struggling and start living*, 2nd edition. Robinson.

Kinman, G. and Teoh, K. (2018) *What could make a difference to the mental health of UK doctors? A review of the research evidence*. Society of Occupational Medicine.

Kroenke, K., Spitzer, R.L. and Williams, J.B. (2001) The PHQ-9: validity of a brief depression severity measure. *J Gen Intern Med*, **16(9):** 606–13.

Kübler-Ross, E. (1970) *On Death and Dying*. Collier Books/Macmillan Publishing Co.

Martell, C.R., Addis, M.E. and Jacobson, N.S. (2001) *Depression in Context: strategies for guided action*. Norton.

Murphy, I.J. (2014) Self-reported and employer-recorded sickness absence in doctors. *Occup Med*, **64(6):** 417–20.

NICE (2018) *Post-traumatic stress disorder* [NG116].

NICE (2022a) *Depression in adults: treatment and management* [NG222].

NICE (2022b) *Mental wellbeing at work* [NG212].

Riley, R., Spiers, J., Buszewicz, M. *et al.* (2018) What are the sources of stress and distress for general practitioners working in England? A qualitative study. *BMJ Open*, **8**:e017361.

Riley, R., Spiers, J., Chew-Graham, C.A. *et al.* (2018) 'Treading water but drowning slowly': what are GPs' experiences of living and working with mental illness and distress in England? A qualitative study. *BMJ Open*, **8(5):**e018620.

Stroebe, M. and Schut, H. (1999) The dual process model of coping with bereavement: rationale and description. *Death Studies*, **23(3):** 197–224.

Uphoff, E., Ekers, D., Robertson, L. *et al.* (2020) Behavioural activation therapy for depression in adults. *Cochrane Database of Systematic Reviews*, **6:** 7(7).

Walker, B., Moss, C., Gibson, J. *et al.* (2019) *Tenth National GP Worklife Survey*. Policy Research Unit in Health and Social Care Systems and Commissioning (PRUComm).

Williams, C. and Garland, A. (2002) A cognitive-behavioural therapy assessment model for use in everyday clinical practice. *Adv Psych Treat,* **8(3):** 172–9.

Worden, J.W. (2009) *Grief Counselling and Grief Therapy: a handbook for the mental health practitioner*, 4th edition. Routledge.

World Health Organization (2019) *International Statistical Classification of Diseases and Related Health Problems*, 11th edition. https://icd.who.int/

Zigmond, A.S. and Snaith, R.P. (1983) The hospital anxiety and depression scale. *Acta Psychiatr Scand*, **67(6):** 361–70.

Support for health professionals

BMA counselling service: free and confidential 24/7 counselling and peer support service open to all doctors and medical students (regardless of BMA membership), plus their partners and dependants.
www.bma.org.uk/advice/work-life-support/your-wellbeing/counselling-and-peer-support

NHS coaching support:
www.england.nhs.uk/supporting-our-nhs-people/support-now/looking-after-you-confidential-coaching-and-support-for-the-primary-care-workforce/

NHS Practitioner Health: a free, confidential NHS primary care mental health and addiction service with expertise in treating health and care professionals.
www.practitionerhealth.nhs.uk/

NHS support for diverse colleagues: coaching and wellbeing support for ethnic minority NHS staff.
www.england.nhs.uk/supporting-our-nhs-people/support-now/support-for-our-diverse-colleagues/

Samaritans: free, 24/7 emotional support service for health and support staff.
Telephone: 116 123
www.samaritans.org/how-we-can-help/contact-samaritan/

Shout 85258 text support: free, 24/7 mental health text support in the UK. Members of the public can access by texting the word SHOUT to 85258; healthcare professionals can text FRONTLINE to the same number (a service contracted out by NHS England) (https://giveusashout.org/)

Support services via NHS England:
www.england.nhs.uk/supporting-our-nhs-people/support-now/

Tea and Empathy: Facebook support group for NHS staff:
www.facebook.com/groups/1215686978446877/